DRUGS

NATURAL

ALTERNATIVES

• •

A Guide to the Uses and Effects of
the Top Prescription Drugs and
Natural Products

CLELL M. FOWLES, PHARMACIST

For orders or information, please contact:

DAC Health
138 East 12300 South, Ste. C #183
Draper, Utah
84020-7965

Disclaimer

The information compiled in this book are based upon the research and the personal and professional experiences of the author. The information contained in this book is for educational purposes only and is not recommended as a means of diagnosing or treating an illness. All matters concerning physical and mental health should be supervised by a health practitioner knowledgeable in treating that particular condition. The author does not prescribe any remedies or assume any responsibility for those who choose to treat themselves.

ISBN 0-9711407-0-7

Contents

Dedication

This book is dedicated to my wife, Debi, and our three children: Sara, Gabryel and Noah. Without their support this book could not have been written.

My thanks also to the many others that have contributed in some way to making this book come true. Thank you!

Foreword

High costs for health insurance, prescription drugs, p
cian services, and health care, in general, have angere
American consumer and spurred the search for self care
natives. The high incidence of adverse drug reactions (
among hospitalized patients resulting in 106,000 death
year: see Lazarou et al., *JAMA*, 279, 1200-1205, 1998) have
thermore, created a questioning distrust of the pharmace
industry and of FDA approved prescription and over
counter drugs. These events have coincided with an incr
since 1994 after the passage of DSHEA, in the availabili
nutritional supplements whose natural sources of origin
clude many of the dangers of synthetic, single-entity, drug
a result, the American consumer now has some intere
choices: to continue with regular drugs as usual, to con
supplements with regular drugs, or to switch to herbal
ucts for all but the most serious of conditions and illn
Significant levels of savings and safety are being accrued
increased use of such herbals, while more and more d
accumulating, as to their safety and efficiency, in our p
sional and scientific journals.

Pharmacist and herb specialist, Clell Fowles, has com
his expertise about today's top prescription drug categ
with his knowledge of herbal products, to create this

Through the past 15 years, Clell has answered thousands of questions and delivered dozens of lectures on herbal supplements. This book will be especially informative to the lay public as they shift more and more to a do-it-yourself approach to health care and maintenance. However, health care professionals, themselves, will also find it helpful as they attempt to learn more about herbal products, their applications, merits, and potential complications, especially when interacting with prescription medications. Clell has avoided the use of many technical terms, and the book is easily understood without the use of a medical dictionary. The book is readable as well as useful and informative.

Jerry L. McLaughlin, Ph.D.
Emeritus Professor of Pharmacognosy
Purdue University

■ CHAPTER 1 ■

Introduction

Writing this book has been a labor of love. My schooling and background is as a pharmacist. This came about because of a love of science and a desire to help people. Through the years I have practiced many forms of pharmacy: nuclear medicine, retail, hospital and home health. Presently I work with natural products and, more specifically, health and safety concerns and drug interactions.

Because of my involvement with natural products, I have become acutely aware of a need for a book such as this. Daily I am asked questions about drug/herb interactions and what nutritional supplement recommendations I have for a person on a certain prescription medication. I have become aware of the fact that many people do not know what their prescription medications are for or what kind of supplements they can use with their prescriptions. That is the point at which this book is addressed.

The scope of the book is to cover the top prescriptions in the United States and herbal and nutritional supplements that may be used for the same conditions. The prescriptions chosen for inclusion are the top selling prescription medications in the United States. There are several thousand prescription medications available, but that is a little too much to cover. Instead I decided that the top selling prescription medications would cover the most ground. Many people are on these prescriptions and many you will have seen on television commercials in spots called "direct to consumer" advertising. These types of commercials allow pharmaceutical companies to market their prescription medications directly to the market for the medication. The caveat, of course, is that you must see your physician for a prescription in order to obtain the medication.

The sections covering prescription medications will list the prescription's brand name, generic name, most common uses and side effects for those medications. Since many medications have the same functions, they are discussed in groups depending upon the medication's pharmacology (actions and properties of the drugs).

Following the information about the drugs comes the section concerning herbals and natural products that may be used for the same indications as the prescriptions. The list of alternatives to the prescription medications is not an exhaustive list. It is designed, instead, to be a beginning point for an individual to start caring for themselves using natural products. The natural products chosen are all mainstream and have good scientific evidence to back their use.

By tying natural products to the pharmacology of the prescriptions, we are, in essence, taking advantage of the greatest strength of western medicine – diagnosis. When we know how a prescription works then we also know the diagnosis. Then, using that diagnosis, we can apply the wonders of nature to guide us back to better health.

Many times a health problem can be rectified simply by using a natural product. Other times an individual may need to be on several natural products or a combination of natural products and prescriptions. Since many people will be mixing prescription medications with natural products, I have tried to identify known interactions between the two. By using this information we can avoid a potential drug/herb interaction.

I am an advocate of natural products. They were the first

medicines used by man and they still should hold a prominent place in our health care arsenal. I do not, however, recommend that anyone abruptly stop their prescription medications. If you are on a prescription medicine and wish to try an herbal alternative as either a replacement for, or in concert with a prescription medication then I recommend you consult your physician or health care professional. You should do this especially if you intend to stop the prescription medication. There are several reasons for this. First we must make sure that the health effects of the prescription are being met by the natural product. For instance, we wouldn't want a person to stop using a high blood pressure medicine to go on a natural product only to have their high blood pressure go out of control. It could be that the person needs to be on more than one natural product, or a combination of a lower dose of prescription medication and a natural product in order to control their blood pressure. Second, there are some prescriptions that are dangerous if abruptly stopped. Prescription medicines are extremely potent compounds and withdrawing them suddenly can often cause problems. You should consult your pharmacist or physician (preferably the physician that prescribed the medicine) as to how to discontinue the drug safely.

The use and research backing natural products has come a long way in the last few years. Many people have discovered the benefits of helping their health with natural products. I have noticed that, as people begin using natural products, they seem to be in better harmony with their health. My wish would be that this book help an individual towards that harmony.

CHAPTER 2

ADD/ADHD

ADD (Attention Deficit Disorder) and ADHD (Attention Deficit Hyperactivity Disorder) are both relatively new to the field of diagnosis. Forty and fifty years ago these were not recognized as distinct disorders. Forty and fifty years ago these were not recognized as distinct disorders. Many have argued that this is because they didn't exist before our modern existence. This argument states that these disorders have come about due to environmental toxins, refined foods, additives, preservatives, etc.

It should be noted that ADD and ADHD are two separate disorders. They are usually lumped together and simply referred to as ADD. ADD involves an inability to concentrate on the part of the individual. This is not linked with a hyperactivity component. ADHD involves both a lack of concentration and the hyperactivity component.

DRUGS

Adderall (mixed amphetamines)
Dexedrine (dextroamphetamine)
Ritalin (methylphenidate)

All of these medications are classified as CNS (central nervous system) stimulants. These drugs are sometimes prescribed to individuals with narcolepsy (sleeping disorder) and to lose weight (by increasing calories burned and decreasing appetite). It may seem strange to utilize a stimulant for someone suffering ADD/ADHD, but it seems that, in children, these drugs have a paradoxical effect – meaning that they cause a reaction exactly opposite of what we would expect. In other words, when given a stimulant such as Ritalin, an ADD/ADHD child will be calmed and more able to focus.

Common Side-Effects of These Medications

Restlessness
Dizziness
Insomnia
Euphoria
Tremor
Headache
Palpitations
Tachycardia (elevated heart rate)
Elevated blood pressure
Diarrhea
Constipation
Anorexia
Impotence
Dependence

Natural Alternatives

Caffeine – Caffeine can be found in various plants and is found in many drinks. Caffeine is also a CNS stimulant and would, therefore, have some of the same effects as the amphetamines. The addition of the sugar, colors, additives, etc. found in soda water is, however, not recommended.

Ephedrine – Ephedrine can be found in the Chinese plant Ma Huang. Ephedrine, or more precisely, the ephedrine alkaloids, are also CNS stimulants. Ephedrine should be used in a standardized preparation so that the same amount of ephedrine alkaloids is delivered with each dose. Ephedrine alkaloids are most commonly found in weight loss products due to their anorexic effects.

Ginseng – Ginseng (*Panax ginseng*) also contains compounds that stimulate the CNS. This is the reason for the use of ginseng in "energy" products.

B-Vitamins – The B-vitamins are very important in brain chemistry. Any individual with ADD/ADHD should supplement with B-vitamins to make sure that enough vitamins are present for proper brain function.

Ginkgo – Ginkgo (*Ginkgo biloba*) has been shown to increase the amount of blood and oxygen that reaches brain cells. This increased cerebral circulation can go a long way towards helping with ADD/ADHD.

Antioxidants – Antioxidants such as grape seed extract and vitamin C help protect brain cells and nerves from oxidative damage from such things as free radicals, toxins, and pollutants.

Flax Seed Oil – Flax seed oil has many benefits. Flaxseed oil has been shown to lower the risk of death from coronary heart disease. Flax seed oil provides essential fatty acids to the system. Essential fatty acids are very important to the central nervous system and, in particular, the brain. Essential fatty acids allow the nerves to operate more efficiently. Some preliminary studies have shown an improvement in ADD/ADHD children with flax seed oil supplementation alone.

Drug/Natural Product Interactions

Ginseng, caffeine and ephedrine alkaloids, since they are CNS stimulants, should be used with extreme caution with any of the prescription medications listed above for ADD/ADHD. Since all are stimulant in nature, there could be additive effects which could lead to unwanted over-stimulation.

Special Considerations

Adderall, Dexedrine and Ritalin are very potent CNS stimulants. They can, over time, lead to dependency. It is extremely important that these medications not be stopped suddenly. If you are on one of these medications for ADD/ADHD and would like to stop using it, you should contact your physician so that he/she can help you stop the medication without unwanted side effects such as depression.

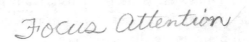

Focus Attention

CHAPTER 3

Allergy Medications

The term "allergy" is broadly used to describe a hypersensitive response to an allergen or antigen. Generally, a person comes into contact with an allergen and becomes sensitized to it. Then, when the person encounters the allergen again, the immune response causes what we typically refer to as an allergy. Allergies can be relatively mild, from sneezing and watery eyes, to quite pronounced, such as anaphylaxis.

Allergies, like many other ailments, seem more prevalent now than they were years ago. This is really not surprising given the fact that the conveniences of our modern society challenge us with many more allergens. Many people suffer from what is termed "seasonal allergies" or "seasonal rhinitis", referring to the stuffy nose and watery eyes that come with an allergic reaction. Other people suffer from year around allergies. These people are usually allergic to different antigens at different times of the year—but the end result is feeling miserable all year long.

Allergies are usually treated with antihistamines. Antihistamines are compounds that block the effects of histamine. Histamine is a compound released by the mast cells in response to an encounter with an allergen. It is the effects of the histamine that cause the watery eyes, itchiness, hives, nasal congestion and so on that are typical of an allergic response.

Alternately, or as adjunct therapy, allergies may be treated with compounds called corticosteroids. These compounds are very potent anti-inflammatory agents and have other, varying, effects on the immune system. For allergies they are usually prescribed as a nasal spray. The corticosteroids are also applied topically (as ointments) for contact dermatitis (a rash on the skin from contact with an allergen such as poison ivy) and as inhalers for the treatment of asthma.

Most allergy medications have the unwanted side effect of pronounced sedation. One common antihistamine, diphenhy- *drug used for treating allergies* dramine (Benadryl), is utilized in many "PM" products due to the sedative effect. The newer antihistamines such as Claritin and Allegra are touted as being much less sedating.

tending to relieve tension

Drugs   *antihistamine*

Claritin (loratadine)
Claritin-D (loratadine and pseudoephedrine)
Seldane (terfenadine)
Allegra (fexofenadine)
Zyrtec (cetirizine)
Flonase (fluticasone)   *Corticosteroids*
Vancenase AQ (beclomethasone)
Beconase AQ (beclomethasone)
Flovent (fluticasone)
Nasonex (mometasone)

Claritin, Claritin-D, Seldane, Allegra and Zyrtec are all classified as antihistamines. Claritin-D combines the antihistamine loratadine with pseudoephedrine. Pseudoephedrine is a mild stimulant, related to ephedrine, which causes constriction of blood vessels. This constriction leads to a decongestant effect, especially in the nose.

Flonase, Vancenase AQ, Beconase AQ, Flovent and Nasonex are all in the corticosteroid category. These products are packaged as a nasal spray to be inhaled directly into the nose. The corticosteroids produce an anti-inflammatory effect on the nasal mucosa (mucous membranes of the nose) and relieve allergies in that way. They also have other effects on the immune system that may change the way in which the immune system responds to an allergen. The net effect is a decrease in the symptoms of an allergic response.

Common Side-Effects of Antihistamines

Drowsiness
Dizziness
Increased appetite
Headache
Weakness
Fatigue
Nervousness
Dry Mouth
Cough
Arthralgia (pain in joints)
Dysmenorrhea (difficult and painful menstruation)
Nausea
Vomiting

Common Side-Effects of the Corticosteroids

Fatigue
Sneezing
Coughing
Localized fungal infections
Headache

DRUGS & NATURAL ALTERNATIVES / 17

Dizziness
Dysmenorrhea (difficult and painful menstruation)
Diarrhea
Edema
Anxiety
Chest pain
Myalgia (muscle pain)
Back pain
Localized irritation
Arthralgia (pain in joints)

Natural Alternatives

Antioxidants – High doses of antioxidants such as grape seed or pine bark (often referred to as OPCs) can help stop an allergic reaction from happening. The OPCs are water-soluble antioxidants, so they have an excellent safety profile. The antioxidant activity stabilizes the mast cells (that contain histamine). This stabilization helps prevent the release of histamine which causes the nasty effects of an allergic reaction.

Bioflavonoids – The bioflavonoids, such as quercitin, are groups of compounds that exhibit antioxidant activity. Quercitin has been used for its reputed effects in reducing the symptoms of allergies. It is believed that this antioxidant activity also helps to stabilize the mast cells. Stabilization of mast cells reduces or prevents the release of histamine which stops or prevents the allergy attack.

Bromelain – Bromelain works as an anti-inflammatory to help control the inflammation that can occur during an allergy attack. Control of the inflammation helps reduce the swelling of the mucous membranes (eyes, throat and nose) during an allergic reaction.

Stinging Nettle – The Stinging Nettle (*Urtica dioica*) leaf has been used for decades to successfully control allergic rhinitis in hay fever sufferers.

Fructus arantia – This fruit contains synephrine, which is a weaker yet longer acting compound similar to ephedrine. Synephrine causes vasoconstriction around the mucous membranes, so it acts as a decongestant to open up the airways and reduce the runny nose and watery eyes.

Ephedrine – Ephedrine, as we discussed earlier, is a relative of pseudoephedrine and is also used as a decongestant.

Cordyceps – Cordyceps is a fungus that reportedly has the effects of opening up air passageways. This could be of benefit to allergy sufferers, especially if they have some asthmatic conditions that accompany their allergy. Cordyceps works quite well at opening up the passageways of the lungs, reversing some of the constriction that can occur during an allergic attack.

Drug/Natural Product Interactions

Both synephrine (from *Fructus arantia*) and ephedrine are stimulants and should be used with caution when taking decongestants such as pseudoephedrine. Too much of this type of stimulant can lead to sleeplessness, anxiety, hypertension, tachycardia (rapid heart rate) and heart palpitations (irregular heartbeats). You should also watch your intake of caffeine if you are taking one of these products since caffeine can also cause this type of stimulation. Look closely at the medication label because pseudoephedrine is often combined with an antihistamine into one product.

Special Considerations

Great care should be taken if you are on an antihistamine. Antihistamines, as we've discussed, are notorious for causing drowsiness. If you start an antihistamine, you should be careful when operating machinery or driving since the drowsiness could interfere.

Hista Block
a L g

■ CHAPTER 4 ■

Angina Medications

Angina is the term that is usually used for the condition known clinically as angina pectoris. This condition refers to a severe constricting pain in the chest that often radiates to the shoulder. It is caused by ischemia (lack of blood flow) to the heart muscle. The ischemia is usually due to coronary disease. Coronary disease is usually attributed to a narrowing of the coronary arteries which supply the heart muscle with blood. During times of stress or exertion these vessels cannot deliver enough blood to the heart to meet the heart's demands. This causes the pressing, constricting, pain called angina.

Drugs

Nitrostat (nitroglycerin)
Monoket (isosorbide mononitrate)
Imdur (isosorbide mononitrate)
Isordil (isosorbide dinitrate)
Sorbitrate (isosorbide dinitrate)
Dilatrate-SR (isosorbide dinitrate)
NitroQuick (nitroglycerin)

These compounds are all nitrates that act as vasodilators. They dilate the coronary vessels that feed blood to the heart muscle. They also dilate other vessels such as vessels in the head. This usually leads to a pronounced headache which occurs after someone has taken a nitrate medication. The coronary artery dilation only lasts for a few hours at most, but this is sufficient time to allow the heart muscle to recover.

The nitrates are the most prescribed class of drug specifically for angina. Other medications could be utilized to help prevent the onset of an angina attack. For instance, Coumadin, which "thins" the blood, could be given to increase blood flow to the heart by preventing blood clot formation. Blood pressure medications could also be given to control blood pressure and stabilize blood flow to the heart. These other medications are discussed in other chapters of this book. This chapter is devoted to those things which can increase blood flow to the heart muscle which is the source of angina.

Common Side-Effects of Nitrates

Tachycardia (rapid heart beat)
Arrhythmias (irregular heart beat)
Hypotension (low blood pressure)
Headache
Apprehension
Weakness
Vertigo (dizziness)
Insomnia
Nightmares
Agitation
Anxiety
Nausea
Urinary Frequency
Arthralgia (joint pain)
Impotence
Diarrhea

Natural Alternatives

Ginkgo – Extracts of the *Ginkgo biloba* plant have been shown slightly to thin the blood and to improve blood vessels which increases blood flow to the brain. These effects can also be seen with blood flow to the heart. Ginkgo is an excellent product to keep sustained blood flow to the heart muscle.

Hawthorn – The berries of the hawthorn plant (*Crataegus oxycantha*) have been used for heart conditions for centuries. The extract of these berries shows an antioxidant effect on the heart and strengthening effects on the heart muscle. In addition, hawthorn may also dilate coronary arteries and help the heart beat more efficiently.

Co-Enzyme Q10 – Co-Enzyme Q10, or CoQ10 (also called ubiquinone), is vital for proper heart function. As people age and have stresses put on them, the levels of CoQ10 decrease. This can lead to problems with the heart including angina. Supplementation with CoQ10 alone has been shown to decrease blood pressure. Anyone with a heart condition, such as angina, or a concern about cardiovascular health should supplement with CoQ10.

Red Clover – The isoflavones in red clover (*Trifolium pratense*) have a heart protective effect and can help improve the elasticity of arteries. This can prevent the onset of angina.

Antioxidants – Antioxidants, especially OPCs (grape seed, pine bark), vitamin E and vitamin C, also help protect the heart and increase elasticity of the arteries, including coronary arteries.

Drug/Natural Product Interactions

Since many of these natural products have many of the same characteristics of nitrates (dilate coronary blood vessels), caution should be used in taking them together. Consult with your physician if you are on a nitrate medication and wish to utilize a natural product to decrease angina and/or decrease the amount of nitrates used.

L - arginine
Ginkgo Hawthorn
Co Q 10 = bring down blood pressure
Cardio Assurance

Brain
Heart   work together
Gums

If you are on this
Coumadin   interacts with everything
                        a theraputic index
don't use
Garlic
Gotu Kola
Ginger
Ginseng

CHAPTER 5

Anxiety Medications

Anxiety is the term used to describe a condition of apprehension of danger and dread. This apprehension is usually accompanied by physical manifestations. Heart rate and blood pressure can increase along with tension and restlessness. Anxiety can be from an immediate situation – this is called an acute anxiety attack. This could be caused by something such as having to give a presentation in front of a large group of people. Anxiety can also be a person's constant companion. These people suffer from chronic anxiety and are constantly in a tense state due to various reasons.

Pharmacologically anxiety is usually treated with a group of compounds called benzodiazepines. The most recognized drug in this group is Valium. The benzodiazepines have varying half-lives (the length of time a drug stays in the body and has pharmacological activity) ranging from many days to just a few hours. The long and medium half-life drugs are usually used for anxiety. Extremely short half-life benzodiazepine drugs are more typically employed as sleep agents (discussed in another chapter).

Drugs
Xanax (alprazolam)
Klonopin (clonazepam)

Ativan (lorazepam)
Buspar (buspirone)
Valium (diazepam)

Xanax, Klonopin, Ativan and Valium are all of the benzodiazepine classification. Valium, Xanax and Ativan are most often prescribed for anxiety conditions. Klonopin is sometimes utilized to treat anxiety, but it is more often prescribed for seizure disorders. Buspar is chemically an azaspirodecanedione, which is chemically and pharmacologically related to the benzodiazepines. It is pharmacologically classified as an anxiolytic (anxiety reducing) drug.

All of these drugs work on the GABA (gamma aminobutyric acid) system. GABA is an important neurotransmitter in the brain. The GABA system is responsible for inhibiting activity in the brain – in other words, it calms the system down. Benzodiazepines act on the GABA system by stimulating GABA receptors, which leads to a calming effect. Many of the benzodiazepines can also lead to a dependency or addiction.

Common Side-Effects of these Medications

Bradycardia (slow heart rate)
Tachycardia (rapid heart rate)
Hypertension
Hypotension
Edema
Sedation
Depression
Lethargy
Fatigue
Lightheadedness
Memory impairment
Confusion

Amnesia
Stupor
Slurred speech
Euphoria
Irritability
Skin rash
Diarrhea
Constipation
Dry mouth
Change in libido
Change in appetite
Visual disturbances
Dependency

Natural Alternatives

Valerian – Valerian (*Valeriana officinalis*) has often been used to help induce sleep. Lower doses, however, can aid in anxiety. Research has shown that extracts of valerian help stimulate the release of GABA in the CNS (central nervous system). Care must be taken to find a dose that will alleviate anxiety without producing too much drowsiness.

Kava Kava – Kava (*Piper methysticum*) is used by the Polynesians as a relaxing drink. Kava will not only calm the central nervous system, but also has an effect on skeletal muscle as a relaxant.

Ginkgo – *Ginkgo biloba* helps increase and improve blood circulation to the brain. This increased blood flow may help some individuals who suffer anxiety, especially chronic anxiety.

Co-Enzyme Q10 – CoQ10 is essential in two areas of the

body in particular – the circulatory system and the brain. Deficiencies of CoQ10 can manifest themselves in many different ways including precipitating anxiety.

B-Vitamins – The B complex vitamins are essential to proper functioning of the brain. Proper nutrition to the brain is an important component of reducing anxiety.

Antioxidants – Antioxidants, such as OPCs (grape seed and pine bark) and vitamin C are excellent at protecting the brain against oxidative damage. Antioxidants may help relieve some anxiety and are a good course of action for CNS health.

Drug/Natural Product Interactions

Extreme caution should be used if mixing Kava Kava or Valerian with any of the benzodiazepines. It would not be too difficult to have an over-sedation since all of these compounds are sedating. In one case, a man, who was taking prescription Xanax, also took Kava Kava and fell into a coma for several days. If you are on a prescription anxiolytic and wish to try one of these natural products, it is strongly suggested that you contact your physician to discontinue the use of the medication properly.

Special Considerations

It cannot be emphasized enough that the anxiolytic medications, as well as kava kava and valerian, can cause drowsiness. Caution should be used when operating machinery or driving while using one of these products. Caution should also be taken in stopping the use of any of the benzodiazepines. Since the benzodiazepines can be habit forming, it is recommended that you contact your physician for advice about stopping your medication. Your physician can help you slowly reduce the dose to minimize the adverse effects of suddenly stopping the medication.

Co Q10

Nutri-Calm

■ CHAPTER 6 ■

Antibiotics/Antifungals/ Antivirals

This category of anti-infectives comprises one of the largest classes of drugs. There are hundreds of different medications to kill bacteria (antibiotics or antibacterials), fungi (antifungals) and viruses (antivirals). The reason so many antibiotics exist is due to resistance. Resistance is a condition wherein an organism, such as bacteria, is exposed to an antibiotic and survive its effects. The bacteria then share this survival information with other bacteria and you end up with the bacteria being resistant to that antibiotic. Medical science then must find a new form of antibiotic to overcome this resistance. The problem of resistance is not a minor concern. Some bacteria are now resistant to the most potent antibiotic created: Vancomycin. Vancomycin resistant strains of bacteria are developing at an alarming rate. If you ask any medical scientist what the most pressing problem of modern medicine is, he will probably reply that it is antibiotic resistance.

This problem has arisen due to many factors. The most common factor is the over prescribing of antibiotics. Antibiotics are routinely given to people with viral infections (antibiotics will not kill viruses), and this process encourages bacteria to become resistant. Another common problem is the fact that many people who are properly prescribed antibiotics do not finish the entire course of therapy. After a few days, they feel much better, so they stop taking the antibiotic. This leads to a sub-therapeutic dose of antibiotic given and allows some of the bacteria (not all of which have been killed since the antibiotic was not finished) to become resistant.

Antibiotics have also created the rise of antifungal medications. Some antibiotics can kill all bacteria, whether friendly bacteria or the invading bacteria. When friendly bacteria are killed there is room for a competing fungus to take over and overgrow. Since there has been a rise in fungal infections, new medications have had to be created to kill the troublesome fungi.

Antiviral medications are a fairly new member of the pharmaceutical family. Man has sought the cure to the common cold for years, but most of the antivirals have been geared towards influenza, Herpes virus, and HIV.

Drugs

Trimox (amoxicillin)
Amoxil (amoxicillin)
Lorabid (loracarbef)
Augmentin (amoxicillin/clavulanate)
Ceclor (cefaclor)
Zithromax (azithromycin)
Pen VK (penicillin)
Cipro (ciprofloxacin)
Keflex (cephalexin)
Septra (sulfamethoxazole/trimethoprim)
Ery Tab (erythromycin)
Ceftin (cefoxitin)
Vibramycin (doxycycline)
Sumycin (tetracycline)
Levaquin (levofloxacin)
Cefzil (cefprozil)

Macrobid (nitrofurantoin)
Floxin (ofloxacin)
Suprax (cefixime)
Duricef (cefadroxil)
Biaxin (clarithromycin)
Bactroban (mupirocin)
Tobradex (tobramycin)
Lotrisone (clotrimazole/betamethasone)
Lamisil (terbinafine)
antifungals
Zovirax (acyclovir)
Diflucan (fluconazole)

Of this list, Lotrisone, Lamisil and Diflucan are antifungals. Zovirax is an antiviral and the rest are antibacterial antibiotics. We could enter into a rather lengthy discussion of the various mechanisms of action of the various antibiotics. It suffices to say, however, that antibiotics work in two basic ways: bacteriostatic (inhibiting the growth and replication of bacteria) and bacteriocidal (actually killing the bacteria). An example of these two types of antibiotics are erythromycin (bacteriostatic) and penicillin (bacteriocidal).

Antifungal medications most commonly destroy the fungus. They do this in a variety of ways, but generally the mechanism involves disrupting the membrane surrounding the fungus. Antivirals work in several different fashions depending on the biochemical nature of the virus. Viruses have many means of infecting and replicating and must be attacked on an individual basis.

Common Side-Effects of these Medications

Allergic reactions
Tachycardia (rapid heart rate)
Hypotension
Vasodilation

Hallucinations
Convulsions
Seizures
Dizziness
Fatigue
Dry Mouth
Insomnia
Drowsiness
Dyspnea (shortness of breath)
Dermatitis (skin inflammation)
Edema
Rash
Nausea
Vomiting
Diarrhea
Fungal infections
Arthralgia (joint pain)
Myalgia (muscle pain)
Asthma
Muscle stiffness
Bradycardia (slow heart rate)
Muscle cramps
Angina (chest pain)
Alteration in taste
Cough
Vertigo
Tinnitis (ringing in ears)
Flushing
Flu-like symptoms

Natural Alternatives

It should be noted that the first antibiotics came from nature. Penicillin was first isolated from a common *Penicillium* fungus. It should also be noted that natural supplements do not offer the extensive variety of anti-infective agents that pharmaceutical science has produced through fermentation, chemical modification, and genetic manipulation. Many new compounds are yet to be discovered in nature, but the pharmaceutical industry has exhaustively searched soil samples for the past fifty years. Nature does offer several unprocessed things, however, to help us if we have a mild infection or to protect us from getting an infection.

Garlic – The active component in garlic, allicin, a sulfur-containing compound has shown activity against various bacteria. Consuming garlic or taking a garlic supplement, in addition to helping with cholesterol and cardiovascular health, can also help ward off an infection. The Russians actually utilized garlic during World War II as an antibiotic when they ran out of penicillin and sulfa drugs, and the ancient Egyptians used garlic extensively as an anti-infective.

Pau D'Arco – Pau D'Arco (*Tabebuia heptaphylla*) contains compounds which have shown activity against bacteria and fungi as well as cancer. There also seems to be some antiviral activity. Many people brew Pau D'Arco into a tea and consume it on a regular basis. This certainly helps them keep away infections that plague their colleagues.

Olive Leaf – Olive leaf (*Olea europea*), which can be purchased as a supplement, has also shown antibacterial and antifungal activity with some antiviral activity. Olive leaf along with garlic proves especially good at fighting infections that occur in the lungs.

Colloidal silver – You can find a colloidal silver solution in many health food stores. This particular solution has silver in solution with a water base. Silver is a very potent antibacterial agent. Silver is used pharmaceutically today in several topical salves that are used on burn patients and others with topical infections. Colloidal silver solutions could also be used topically in this manner by soaking a sterile cloth with the silver solution and applying it to the topical infection. Care should be taken in choosing a company with a good reputation when buying colloidal silver. Many companies simply sell bottled water which is labeled as colloidal silver. This type of situation could actually exacerbate a topical infection since the water is probably not sterile.

Echinacea (*Echinacea spp.*) and Golden Seal (*Hydrastis canadensis*) – Both of these plants have been employed by man to enhance the immune system. Testing has been performed on these compounds and bears out the fact that they do, indeed, boost the immunity. Many people incorporate these two plants as part of a year around defense against invading organisms.

Vitamin C – Much has been discussed about the role of vitamin C in immune function and in infective states. The author will simply say that he has found vitamin C very useful in times of infection.

Zinc – Many companies offer zinc lozenges for use during cold seasons. Several studies have been conducted and have had different outcomes. My personal experience leads me to believe that zinc does play a role in reducing the symptoms and duration of the common cold. The mechanism of action is probably through an interaction between the zinc atom and the cold virus. It is important to note that the zinc lozenge should not be swallowed. The zinc ions seem to exert their activity in the throat and mouth, so the lozenge should be allowed to dissolve slowly in the mouth where the zinc can bind cold virus.

Friendly bacteria (also called "probiotics") – The role of friendly bacteria in warding off an infection should not be overlooked. These friendly bacteria, such as acidophilus and bifidophilus, inhabit our intestinal tracts and could actually be described as part of our immune system. Invading organisms have a harder time getting a foothold if friendly bacteria are competing with them. Daily supplementation with these bacteria can help us reduce the number of infections we have. It should also be noted that antibiotics also kill these friendly bacteria. If you are on an antibiotic, you should supplement with these products to re-establish the friendly bacterial colonies. This will also help reduce the incidence of thrush or other fungal overgrowth infections that are a common side-effect during a course of antibiotic treatment.

L-Lysine – This amino acid has been shown to have positive effects on the immune system. It should be noted that l-lysine seems particularly good at fighting the Herpes Simplex virus (that causes cold sores).

Arabinogalactan and Beta Glucans (1,3/1,6) – These compounds are long-chain polysaccharides that directly stimulate the immune system. They seem to mimic the polysaccharides of bacterial cell walls and capsules, which causes a response from the immune system that increases the production of macrophages, T-cells, B-cells, natural killer cells, cytokines and antibodies.

Caprylic acid – Caprylic acid, which can be isolated from coconut oil, has been shown to have antifungal properties.

Drug/Natural Product Interactions

There are no known interactions between any of these natural products and prescription antibiotics. If you are on an antibiotic you can discontinue the use of the natural product while you're on the drug. Once you have completed a course of antibiotics, it is highly recommend to use a friendly bacterial, probiotic, product to re-establish normal bacterial colonies and reduce the risk of fungal infections.

Special Considerations

Although nature allows us to utilize these products to help protect ourselves against infections, it must be remembered that these products are mild in comparison to the antibiotics. If you have a serious infection, please seek medical advice. If you use these natural products, you will experience fewer infections, but this still won't stop all infections. What nature does allow is fewer infections and milder infections when they do occur.

Nature's Immune Stimulator

■ CHAPTER 7 ■

Antidepressants

Depression is another disorder that has seen a rise in diagnosis, at least from the point of the number of prescriptions written for antidepressants. There could be several reasons for this. It could be that medical science is better at diagnosing such disorders. It is also possible that with today's modern lifestyle, depression occurs more often. It could also be that physicians are simply writing prescriptions for antidepressants whenever they get a patient with vague symptoms and they have no other explanation for their complaint.

Regardless of the cause, pharmacology has been moving constantly forward in developing new antidepressants. The original antidepressants were compounds known as MAOIs (monoamine oxidase inhibitors). These antidepressants, although heralded as a major advance at the time, were crude and came with many side effects. The next generation of antidepressants was the tricyclics. Tricyclic antidepressants were a major step forward from the MAOIs, but they still came with many side effects. The tricyclics are still prescribed quite often today, but the MAOIs are only rarely used.

The next major advance over the tricyclics was the advent of the SSRIs (selective serotonin reuptake inhibitors). The class of drugs known as SSRIs constitutes one of the most heavily prescribed classes of pharmaceuticals. SSRIs will, more than likely, be the drug of choice prescribed for a newly diagnosed case of depression.

Drugs

Prozac (fluoxetine)
Zoloft (sertraline)
Paxil (paroxetine)
Effexor (venlafaxine)
Elavil (amitriptyline)
Wellbutrin (bupropion)
Celexa (citalopram)
Desyrel (trazodone)
Serzone (nefazodone)

Prozac, Paxil, Zoloft and Celexa are all categorized as SSRIs. The SSRIs work by inhibiting the reuptake of the neurotransmitter serotonin. Normally serotonin is released into the synapse (space between two nerve cells) to carry the nervous impulse to the next nerve cell. After its release, serotonin is then taken back up, for reuse, by the nerve cell. SSRIs inhibit the ability of the cell to take up the serotonin. This allows more serotonin to remain in the synapse and, therefore, causes more stimulation. The neurotransmitter serotonin has been shown to have a major impact on most types of depression and is being looked at as a possible contributor to many other disorders.

Effexor and Serzone are both new types of antidepressants that are unrelated to the SSRIs, tricyclics or MAOIs. Their mechanism of action is not completely understood, but they do raise levels of serotonin and norepinephrine by decreasing reuptake of these neurotransmitters.

Elavil and Desyrel are both typical members of the tricyclic antidepressant drugs. Tricyclics also work on blocking reuptake of serotonin and norepinephrine. They also possess other characteristics, such as drowsiness, that have them prescribed for other conditions besides depression. Elavil, for example, has shown some limited benefit for people suffering from certain types of chronic pain.

The MAOIs are hardly ever used anymore. The drugs that make up the class of MAOIs are: Nardil (phenelzine), Parnate (tranylcypromine) and Marplan (isocarboxazid). These medications are usually reserved for individuals with resistant or severe depression.

Common Side-Effects for these Drugs

Hypertension
Hypotension
Abnormal dreams
Agitation
Anxiety
Confusion
Dizziness
Drowsiness
Insomnia
Headache
Hallucinations
Mania
Tremor
Fatigue
Rash
Pruritus (itching)
Edema
Weight loss
Weight gain
Nausea
Vomiting

Increased appetite
Decreased appetite
Myalgia (muscle pain)
Blurred vision
Urinary frequency
Sexual dysfunction
Back pain
Dry mouth
Tinnitis (ringing in ears)
Change in taste perception

Natural Alternatives

B-vitamins – Once again we must not underestimate the powerful effect that B-vitamins have on the central nervous system. The CNS requires B-vitamins for proper functioning. Since B-vitamins are water-soluble, their reserves can be depleted rather quickly. Many patients gain great benefits from supplementation with a B-vitamin complex.

Flax Seed (EFAs) – Flax seed or fish oils are excellent sources of essential fatty acids (EFAs). EFAs are extremely important for proper nerve health. The nerve cells require EFAs in their structure and supplementation with EFAs permits proper and more efficient conduction of nerve impulses through a nerve cell.

Antioxidants – Antioxidants such as the OPCs (i.e., grape seed extract, pine bark extract) and vitamin C are excellent at reducing oxidative damage in the CNS. Antioxidant supplementation is highly recommended for individuals with depression or CNS disorders.

Co-Enzyme Q10 (CoQ10) – CoQ10, as we've discussed before, is very active in the functioning of the CNS. Reserves of

CoQ10 can be depleted quickly, so CoQ10 supplementation is recommended for good CNS health.

Ginkgo – *Ginkgo biloba* increases the blood flow to the CNS. Often this helps alleviate symptoms of depression by supplying proper blood supply to the brain. Ginkgo has also been shown to help with memory through this same mechanism.

Ginseng – Ginseng (*Panax ginseng*) has been used for centuries to increase energy. For people with depression this is sometimes the answer.

Ephedrine – Oftentimes depression is not the problem. Fatigue or lack of energy is often confused with depression. Ephedrine containing products can aid in reducing fatigue for individuals with this condition.

St. John's Wort – The *Hypericum perforatum* plant has been utilized by man for centuries to alleviate depression. Generally St. John's Wort is safe and effective for mild to moderate depression. The mechanism of action of St. John's Wort is not clearly understood, but it seems to raise dopamine, serotonin and norepinephrine levels in the CNS.

SAM-e – SAM-e (pronounced "sammy") stands for S-adenosylmethionine. This substance is naturally occurring in the body and provides a methyl group (-CH3) for chemical reactions. The body utilizes methyl groups to form new compounds such as neurotransmitters. SAM-e has undergone extensive testing in Europe where it has been shown to raise levels of neurotransmitters in the CNS. It is also believed that SAM-e may help the nerve cells increase their efficiency by providing the rebuilding blocks for nerve repair. Regardless of its mechanism of action, SAM-e shows great promise as a natural product for individuals suffering from depression. SAM-e tablets must be enteric coated and taken on an empty stomach. This is because the SAM-e can react in the stomach to food and stomach acid, which greatly reduce the amount absorbed and delivered to the CNS.

Drug/Natural Product Interactions

Ephedrine and ginseng should not be used with monoamine oxidase inhibitors (MAOIs) due to the potential for overstimulation.

St. John's Wort has been shown to have an interaction with two different medications: Sandimmune (cyclosporine – an anti-rejection drug for transplants) and Crixivan (indinavir – an antiviral agent used in HIV infections). In both of these circumstances, the St. John's Wort changes the blood levels of the drug. If you are on either of these medications, you should consult your physician before taking St. John's Wort.

There is a theoretical interaction between SAM-e and any of the antidepressants. Clinically no interaction has been shown, but care should be taken if an antidepressant is currently being used and SAM-e supplementation is being considered.

Special Considerations

The antidepressants are very potent compounds. You should discuss their use with your physician and be aware of the potential side-effects. Suddenly stopping an antidepressant is not recommended. Many of these antidepressants have effects that could create a withdrawal syndrome if suddenly discontinued. If you are on an antidepressant and wish to try a natural alternative, please consult your physician.

■ CHAPTER 8 ■

Asthma Medications

Asthma, as with many of the other ailments we've discussed, seems to have increased in prevalence in the last few decades. This could easily be due to the increase in pollutants and other allergens and toxins in the air. Asthma usually affects children, but can also be seen in adults.

The term asthma used to denote any case of difficult breathing. Now it is used to denote the condition known as bronchial asthma. Asthma is a condition of the lungs in which there is a generalized narrowing (constriction) of the airways. This is associated with spasm of smooth muscle, edema of the mucosa and accumulation of mucous. The changes in lung functioning are a result of the local release of spasmogens and other substances such as histamine, leukotrienes and prostaglandins.

Asthma can be treated with various kinds of medications. Most commonly a drug is inhaled into the lungs which has the direct effect of relaxing smooth muscle and opening up the lung passageways. Asthma is also treated with inhaled corticosteroids, which act to reduce the swelling and buildup of mucous. Some newer medications work on the prostaglandins or leukotrienes that play a part in an asthma attack.

Drugs

Vanceril (beclomethasone)
Beconase (beclomethasone)
Proventil (albuterol)
Atrovent (ipratropium)
Serevent (salmeterol)
Azmacort (triamcinolone)
Singulair (montelukast)
Combivent (ipratropium/albuterol)
Accolate (zafirlukast)
Alupent (metaproterenol)
Tornalate (bitolterol)
Isuprel (isoproterenol)
Brethine (terbutaline)
Pulmicort (budesonide)
AeroBid (flunisolide)

Azmacort, Pulmicort, AeroBid, Beconase and Vanceril are all classified as corticosteroids. These medications decrease the swelling and mucous buildup associated with asthma. Corticosteroids for the treatment of asthma, such as these listed here, are all inhaled. Physicians will sometimes prescribe oral medications, such as prednisone, that also reduce swelling.

Singulair and Accolate are both leukotriene receptor antagonists. They take advantage of the role of leukotrienes in asthma. By blocking these receptors, many of the manifestations of asthma are stopped or reduced.

Proventil, Atrovent, Isuprel, Alupent, Tornalate, Serevent, Combivent and Brethine are all broadly classified as bronchodilators. These work directly to relax smooth muscle. The passageways of the lungs are comprised of smooth muscle. During an asthma attack, this smooth muscle constricts, reducing the airflow in the lungs. By relaxing the smooth muscle in the lungs, airflow can be re-established.

Common Side-Effects of these Medications

Palpitations (irregular heart beat)
Tachycardia (rapid heart beat)
Hypertension
Chest tightness
Weakness
Drowsiness
Restlessness
Insomnia
Headache
Nausea
Vomiting
Diarrhea
Dry Mouth
Flushing
Sweating
Cough
Rash
Dizziness
Joint pain
Back pain
Change in taste perception
Infection
Fever

Natural Alternatives

Bee Pollen – Bee pollen is actually an allergen. Many practitioners of natural medicine have used bee pollen orally to build up immunity to one of the causative agents for asthma. This would be much the same as taking allergen shots to build up immunity and prevent future asthma or allergy attacks. This course of therapy has proven effective for some individuals.

Antioxidants – As discussed in the chapter on allergies, we know that antioxidants can stabilize mast cells which release histamine. The effect of antioxidants goes beyond just mast cells and histamine. Antioxidants may help stabilize several of the processes which can lead to an asthma attack. Antioxidant therapy could help to reduce the occurrence and severity of asthma attacks.

Synephrine – The active ingredient of orange peel, synephrine, acts as a sympathomimetic. This means that it would have the effect of a bronchodilator. Keeping the passageways of the lungs dilated will keep air moving through the lungs and slow or stop an asthma attack.

Ephedrine – Ephedrine is also a bronchodilator. Just like synephrine, its effects are as a sympathomimetic. Ephedrine will also relax smooth muscle in the lungs to dilate the bronchioles and help keep air flowing.

Cordyceps – Cordyceps is a fungus that has been used for several different reasons. Cordyceps has the effect of relaxing smooth muscle and has been shown to help open up air passageways in the lungs. Many asthma sufferers have found varying degrees of relief through supplementation with cordyceps. This natural product may decrease the severity and frequency of asthma attacks.

Drug/Natural Product Interactions

The bronchodilator medications should be used with caution with synephrine and ephedrine due to the possibility of overstimulation.

Special Considerations

Asthma can be a life threatening condition. It is advised that your physician be informed of any proposed changes in your asthma therapy by the addition of natural products. These natural products can be quite effective, but drugs may still have to be utilized to treat this disorder properly.

Lobelia
Hista Block
a Lg

CHAPTER 9

Cholesterol

During the last few decades cholesterol has become a hot topic. We have known for some time that cholesterol is essential as the backbone for hormone production. We now know, however, that a high cholesterol level (usually defined as above 200 mg/dl) is detrimental to cardiovascular health. Cholesterol can be a contributing factor to plaque buildup in the arteries of the circulatory system. This buildup can lead to a number of problems with the circulatory system, so it is imperative that a healthy cholesterol level be maintained. Diet and exercise are often prescribed for this condition, but sometimes levels are high enough that, even with diet and exercise, some other means must be employed to regulate the cholesterol levels.

Drugs

Lopid (gemfibrozil)
Zocor (simvastatin)
Mevacor (lovastatin)
Pravachol (pravastatin)
Lescol (fluvastatin)
Lipitor (atorvastatin)

Zocor, Mevacor, Pravachol, Lescol and Lipitor (commonly referred to as the "statins") are all classified as inhibitors of 3-hydroxy-3-methylglutaryl-coenzyme A (HMG-CoA) reductase (or, HMG-CoA reductase inhibitors). HMG-CoA reductase is an enzyme that converts HMG-CoA to mevalonate. This conversion occurs early in the synthesis of cholesterol and is the rate-limiting step in the synthesis of cholesterol. Therefore, if we inhibit the activity of the enzyme HMG-CoA reductase, we reduce the amount of cholesterol the body produces. This has proven to be a very effective means of controlling cholesterol levels.

Lopid (gemfibrozil) is another drug often prescribed for people with high cholesterol levels. Lopid does not work as an HMG-CoA reductase inhibitor. The exact mechanism of action of Lopid isn't known, but it is known to increase HDL cholesterol (the "good" cholesterol) levels and decrease serum cholesterol levels.

Common Side-Effects for this class of Drugs

Headache
Dizziness
Insomnia
Nausea/Vomiting
Diarrhea
Constipation
Heartburn
Dry Mouth
Leg pain
Shoulder pain
Myalgia (pain in a muscle)
Back pain
Chest pain
Rash

Fatigue
Blurred vision
Cough
Arthralgia (severe pain in a joint)

Natural Alternatives

Red Rice – Several companies now offer a product made from the fermentation of red rice (*Monascus purpureus*). This fermentation process has been shown to produce low levels of compounds similar to the "statin" medications that we've already discussed. The red rice product produces an HMG-CoA reductase inhibition that, as we have seen, decreases cholesterol synthesis. These various red rice products are quite effective at reducing total cholesterol and LDL (bad cholesterol) levels. This choice would be especially beneficial to individuals who are borderline high in their cholesterol readings. Since the red rice product contains actives that are like those of the "statin" drugs, it is not recommended that they be taken together without your doctor's consent.

Garlic – Garlic has been utilized as a food flavoring agent for centuries. It has been recently discovered that garlic exhibits a non-specific mechanism of action to reduce cholesterol levels and LDL levels. Using about 1-2 cloves of fresh garlic daily in flavoring meals will go a long way to promoting healthy cholesterol. The use of a garlic supplement is also effective at achieving these goals. In choosing a supplement, beware of "deodorized" garlic products. The active ingredient in garlic, allicin, is also the part which produces the characteristic garlic odor. Many supplements remove the allicin to make a "deodorized" product, and, in so doing, also remove the beneficial ingredient. Garlic can safely be used with the cholesterol prescription medications we've talked about. Adding garlic to a cholesterol medication could reduce the dose or need for the cholesterol medication.

Fiber – Products such as psyllium and psyllium hulls add fiber to the diet. Not only is this healthy in providing bulk for the intestinal system, it also reduces cholesterol. Cholesterol is secreted into the intestinal system through the gall bladder along with and as part of the bile salts. Further down the intestinal system these materials are reabsorbed. Fiber can effectively bind the cholesterol and bile salts in the intestinal system and remove them with the additional waste. Cholesterol must then be converted by the liver into new bile salts. Supplementation with a fiber product can, thus, produce a significant lowering of cholesterol levels. This is something that can easily be incorporated into a cholesterol-healthy diet and with cholesterol lowering drugs. Care should be taken to consume plenty of water with a high fiber product. You should also space the time you take medications or supplements to not coincide with the fiber product, since the fiber product could also remove part of the medication or supplement. Fiber supplements can be found as capsules, pills and drink mixes. A fiber supplement can also decrease your use of cholesterol medication. In some cases, fiber supplementation is all that is required to reduce cholesterol to normal levels.

Drug/Natural Product Interactions

The red rice compound should not be taken with any of the "statin" medications since they work in the same way. If you are interested in trying one of the red rice products, and you are already on a "statin" medication, then you should consult your physician.

Special Considerations

The "statin" medications, including the red rice products (but to a lesser degree since the level of activity in red rice doesn't compare to the prescriptions) have been shown to decrease reserve levels of Co-Enzyme Q10 (CoQ10) in the body. CoQ10 is essential for energy production, cardiac health, and brain functioning. If you are on a "statin" medication it would be recommended that you supplement with about 100 milligrams of CoQ10 per day. CoQ10 is a water-soluble compound, so the possibility of overdose is slight. Supplementing with 100 milligrams of CoQ10 per day will help keep the stores of CoQ10 in the body adequate during "statin" drug use.

Loclo
Psyllium
Fat Grabbers
Omega 3
Flaxseed
Lecithin

CHAPTER 10

Diabetic Medications

Diabetes is a disorder affecting the utilization of sugar by the body. The condition concerns both the amount of insulin and the effect that insulin has on cells. The net effect is that the cells do not properly utilize glucose, which is fuel for the cells. Diabetes, if left uncontrolled, can have many long-term effects on many body systems.

There are two general classifications of diabetes: type I and type II. Type I diabetes formerly was referred to as juvenile onset diabetes or insulin dependent diabetes. In type I diabetes there is a problem with the pancreas and the ability of the pancreas to produce insulin. Type I diabetics require insulin injections on a regular basis to control their blood sugar.

Type II diabetes, commonly referred to as adult onset diabetes, is a condition that has risen in prevalence the last few decades. This is due to the increasing incidence of obesity in our modern lifestyles. Obesity can lead to cell insulin receptor resistance. This resistance to insulin prevents the cell from taking in blood glucose. Type II diabetics often take oral medication which helps the cells accept insulin and permit glucose entry. These drugs are called oral hypoglycemics. Type II diabetics may or may not require insulin injections since their ability to produce insulin is generally not compromised and is not the problem.

Drugs

Glucophage (metformin)
Glucotrol (glipizide)
Glynase (glyburide)
Rezulin (troglitazone)
Amaryl (glimepiride)
Humulin (human insulin)
Novolin (human insulin)
Diabinese (chlorpropamide)
Tolinase (tolazamide)
Micronase (glyburide)

Humulin and Novolin are two types of human insulin for injection. The insulin is actually produced by genetically altered bacteria. Prior to human insulin for injection, injectable insulin came from the pancreas glands of pigs and cattle. Human insulin has greatly reduced the incidence of adverse reactions associated with pig and cattle insulin injections.

All the other medications are considered oral hypoglycemics. They have different subdivisions, but they all reduce blood sugar. Generally, they work by reducing the resistance to insulin at the insulin receptor sites of cells or by promoting insulin release from sluggish pancreatic cells. This allows the insulin to stimulate the cell to take up glucose. These types of medication have proven to be very effective in controlling type II diabetes. Some of the newer oral hypoglycemics work by stimulating insulin production in the pancreas or lowering the amount of glucose released from the liver.

It should be noted that Rezulin (troglitazone) has been withdrawn from the market in the United States. This was due to a series of serious adverse events that resulted in several deaths. Rezulin is mentioned here due to the fact that it was one of the most prescribed drugs, appearing on the list of top prescribed medications that was used to assemble this book.

Common Side-Effects of Oral Hypoglycemics

Hypoglycemia (low blood sugar)
Blood disorders
Drowsiness
Nervousness
Tremor
Fatigue
Dizziness
Headache
Decreased libido
Vertigo
Chills
Confusion
Diarrhea
Taste alteration
Constipation
Tinnitus (ringing in ears)
Liver function abnormalities
Blurred vision

Natural Alternatives

Ginseng – Ginseng (*Panax ginseng*) has been shown in a few studies to have a blood sugar lowering effect. The exact mechanism of action for this is not known, but it does have the potential to help control blood sugar.

Gymnema – *Gymnema sylvestre* has also been utilized to help control blood sugar. This plant also has experimentally shown the ability to lower blood sugar. This is probably done in the same way most of the oral hypoglycemics work – by changing the sensitivity of insulin receptors to insulin.

Fenugreek – Fenugreek (*Trigonella foenum-graecum*) has been used to treat diabetes because it also lowers blood sugar and has an antioxidant effect. The antioxidant effect is quite beneficial since the disease of diabetes can cause so much destruction due to oxidative actions. The antioxidant effect would help protect against some of that oxidative destruction.

Chromium – The element chromium has a role in diabetes. Deficiencies of chromium have resulted in insulin resistance and high blood sugar. It is evident that chromium is essential to maintain proper blood sugar levels. Supplementation with chromium has been shown to lower blood sugar in diabetic patients.

Bitter Melon – The bitter melon (*Momordica charantia*) has also been used extensively to treat diabetes. It has an effect similar to gymnema and lowers blood sugar by altering the insulin receptor's sensitivity to insulin.

Banaba leaf – The leaf of the banaba (*Lagerstroemia speciosa*), as with the other plants mentioned, has also been used in cases of diabetes. Banaba acts as a hypoglycemic, probably by working on the insulin receptors to promote glucose transport into cells.

Bilberry – Bilberry (*Vaccinium myrtillus*) is mentioned because of its excellent antioxidant activity. Bilberry seems especially good at protecting against the oxidative action in the eyes of diabetic patients. Diabetics often suffer from a condition known as diabetic retinopathy that, over time, will destroy the retina of the eye. Bilberry seems particularly good at protecting the eye against this particular type of retinopathy.

Nopal – Nopal (*Opuntia streptacantha*), also called prickly pear cactus provides nutrients for the liver and aids in digestion and maintaining blood sugar levels. The ability of nopal to lower blood sugar is well documented. This may occur because of its action on the liver. The liver is an important source of blood sugar, as demonstrated by some of the newer oral hypoglycemics which exert their action on the liver.

Drug/Natural Product Interactions

Diabetes is a serious condition and should be appropriately treated. If you are a diabetic and on insulin or an oral hypoglycemic, you should consult your physician if you wish to try a natural product which lowers blood sugar. If the blood sugar is lowered too much it can cause a life-threatening situation. Care should be taken to monitor blood sugars when starting one of these natural products. Your physician can recommend ways of lowering the dose of oral hypoglycemic that you are using if the natural product begins working for you. Your physician can also direct you on insulin dosing and about lowering your insulin dosage appropriately if the natural product is successful at reducing your blood sugar.

Special Considerations

It is highly recommended that any person suffering diabetes take a bilberry supplement for the antioxidant effect. Other antioxidants are also recommended in addition to the bilberry. Antioxidant supplementation may be undertaken without consideration to the blood sugar or any medication use. But it should be noted that blood sugars should be monitored close-ly anytime some new drug or supplement is added to the daily regimen.

treatment

$$\eta BS - a \checkmark$$

Sugar—Reg

CHAPTER 11

Diuretics

Diuretics are a class of pharmaceuticals that increase the amount of urine produced. Diuretics are used for many different reasons. Sometimes a person is simply holding too much water (edema). For a person with edema, diuretics help remove the water which usually accumulates in the lower extremities (legs and ankles).

The diuretics are also often used for individuals with hypertension (high blood pressure). Diuretics remove excess fluid which then lowers the amount of pressure required by the heart to move blood to all the extremities. Diuretics are often the first line of prescriptions offered to a newly diagnosed hypertensive patient. They have proven quite effective at reducing blood pressure in hypertensive individuals. Oftentimes the diuretics will be combined with another antihypertensive to get a better response.

Drugs

Lasix (furosemide) *Loop diuretics*
Maxzide (triamterene/hydrochlorothiazide)
Dyazide (triamterene/hydrochlorothiazide)
Diuril (chlorothiazide)
Oretic (hydrochlorothiazide) *Thiazide diuretics*
HCTZ

Enduron (methyclothiazide)
Lozol (indapamide)
Zaroxolyn (metolazone)
Hygroton (chlorthalidone)
Bumex (bumetanide)   *Loop diuretics*
Demadex (torsemide)
Aldactone (spironolactone)   *Potassium sparing diuretics*

Lasix, Bumex and Demadex are all classified as loop diuretics. These are the most powerful diuretics and have the potential to cause a very serious side effect – hypokalemia (low potassium levels). If the dose of one of these medications is high enough, the physician will usually also have the patient take a potassium supplement. Low blood potassium levels can

lowering blood pressure

Aldactone and triamterene (in Maxzide and Dyazide) are classified as potassium sparing. *Lizzie* They have a weak diuretic effect but are often added to the potassium

Hydrochlorothiazide these diuretics are used with other potassium diuretics or loop diuretics to decrease the amount of potassium

Zaroxolyn, Lozol, Enduron, Oretic and Diuril are all from the class of diuretics known as thiazide diuretics. The thiazides increase the amount of sodium and chloride excreted from the kidney. They will also decrease potassium levels, but not nearly to the degree caused by the loop diuretics.

Common Side-Effects of Diuretics

Hypotension
Dizziness
Vertigo
Headache
Weakness

Restlessness
Insomnia
Anxiety
Depression
Blurred vision
Anorexia
Nausea
Vomiting
Diarrhea
Constipation
Nocturia (need to urinate at night)
Fever
Rash
Dry mouth
Electrolyte imbalance
Muscle cramps

Natural Alternatives

There are many plants that have active ingredients with diuretic effects. Following are but a few with which the author has had personal experience. Please consult an herbalist for a more complete list of plants with diuretic effects. One plant source may be better for your particular condition than another.

Uva Ursi – The uva ursi (*Arctostaphylos uva-ursi*) plant has shown to be a fairly effective diuretic and urinary antiseptic. Use of the plant as a diuretic dates back many centuries.

Buchu – As with uva ursi, the buchu (*Barosma spp.*) has proven itself a useful diuretic.

Nettle – Nettle (*Urtica dioica*) has a history of use as a diuretic. Nettle, buchu and uva ursi are all traditionally utilized for various conditions involving the urinary tract. This is due to their diuretic ability.

Dandelion – The dandelion (*Taraxacum officinale*) has proven particularly effective as a diuretic. Utilizing the dandelion can have many of the same effects as the prescription diuretics.

Golden Rod – Golden Rod (*Solidago virgaurea*), like dandelion, is also a very effective diuretic. Both plants have been utilized to reduce blood pressure and to alleviate swelling and edema. Both have proven very useful.

cranberry/buchu Concentrate Urinary System

Drug/Natural Product Interactions

Care should be exerted when combining a natural diuretic with a prescription diuretic. Combining the actions of these diuretics could potentiate an over-diuresis. Too much diuretic action could lead to electrolyte imbalances and other problems. Consult a health care professional before combining diuretics.

Special Considerations

If you are being treated with a diuretic or believe that a diuretic is appropriate for your condition, please consult a health care professional to ensure that the underlying condition is being addressed. Diuretics are prescribed for conditions such as hypertension and other conditions that cause edema. If you are in this situation, you should make sure the hypertension or other condition is being considered and treated. Nature offers many excellent diuretics and one may offer you the benefits for which you are searching.

CHAPTER 12

High Blood Pressure

Hypertension, also known as high blood pressure, is a disorder that afflicts millions of individuals – with new cases diagnosed each year. High blood pressure can be hard to treat. Headache is sometimes a sign, but many times the disease has few manifestations. The treatment often makes an individual feel worse than any effects they have from the high blood pressure.

We know, however, that high blood pressure should be treated to minimize the unwanted effects which high blood pressure will cause. High blood pressure contributes to many different ailments such as hardening of the arteries, stroke, senility in later life, blindness, and heart disease to name a few. Treating high blood pressure keeps all of our body systems in better shape. We have a much better chance of living a long and healthy life if we keep our blood pressure in check.

Knowing the extremely important role that high blood pressure plays in our health, the pharmaceutical industry has created ever-advancing modes to treat it. There are many different systems that affect our blood pressure and the drugs are designed around those many systems. Often, however, the patient has to try several different drugs before controlling his/her hypertension, this is probably due to the multiple etiologies (causes) that are possible.

Drugs

Vasotec (enalapril)
Procardia (nifedipine)
Calan (verapamil)
Capoten (captopril)
Cardizem (diltiazem)
Tiazac (diltiazem)
Norvasc (amlodipine)
Zestril (lisinopril)
Prinivil (lisinopril)
Tenormin (atenolol)
Toprol (metoprolol)
Lopressor (metoprolol)
Cardura (doxazosin)
Accupril (quinapril)
Hytrin (terazosin)
Ziac (bisoprolol/hydrochlorothiazide)
Monopril (fosinopril)
Cozaar (losartan)
Lotensin (benazepril)
Adalat (nifedipine)
Diovan (valsartan)
Hyzaar (losartan/hydrochlorothiazide)
Inderal (propranolol)
Altace (ramipril)
Plendil (felodipine)
Catapres (clonidine)
Avapro (irbesartan)
Lotrel (amlodipine/benazepril)
Atacand (candesartan)

*Also see the chapter on diuretics. Diuretics are often used to decrease blood pressure because they lower the amount of blood volume, lower the strain on the heart, and, consequently, decrease blood pressure.

Hypertension often requires therapy with more than one agent. Many of the antihypertensive medications combine two ingredients together. Examples of these are Ziac, Hyzaar and Lotrel. Ziac combines a beta-blocking agent with a diuretic. Hyzaar combines an ACE inhibitor with a diuretic. Lotrel combines two different ACE inhibitors. (These various classifications are described below).

Vasotec, Capoten, Zestril, Prinivil, Accupril, Monopril, Atacand, Cozaar, Lotensin, Diovan and Altace all work on the renin-angiotensin system. Renin is a substance that is produced by the kidneys. Renin is converted into angiotensin I which is then converted into angiotensin II. Angiotensin II is a very potent compound that causes vasoconstriction. This increases blood pressure. Angiotensin II also stimulates the secretion of aldosterone from the adrenal cortex. Aldosterone adds to sodium and fluid retention which increases the load on the heart and raises blood pressure.

The enzyme responsible for the conversion of renin to angiotensin I and for angiotensin I to angiotensin II is called angiotensin converting enzyme. These medications work to inhibit the actions of this enzyme. By inhibiting angiotensin converting enzyme, angiotensin II and aldosterone are not formed or released. This causes a considerable decrease in blood pressure. These drugs are referred to as angiotensin converting enzyme inhibitors or ACE inhibitors (also called ACEIs). The ACE inhibitors have become very popular in treating hypertension. A newer class is exemplified by Cozaar and Atacand which block the vascular receptors for angiotensin II.

Tenormin, Toprol, Lopressor and Inderal are all classified as beta-blockers. Beta receptors are found in the heart and cardiovascular system. Blocking these beta sites causes a slowing of the sinus heart rate. This decreases cardiac output and blood pressure. Because of their actions on heart rate, beta-blockers are often prescribed for other indications besides hypertension.

Procardia, Calan, Cardizem, Norvasc, Adalat and Plendil are all from a class of drug referred to as calcium channel blockers. Calcium channels are found in specialized conducting cells in the heart. Blocking these channels forces the heart to beat slower with more time between beats to allow more blood to fill the ventricles. The overall effect is a slower heart rate with a more efficient beat. This also leads to a decrease in blood pressure. Calcium channel blockers, like the beta-blockers, will often be prescribed for conditions besides hypertension due to their actions on heart rate.

Cardura, Hytrin and Catapres are classified as adrenergic agents. Catapres acts centrally (within the CNS) to stimulate alpha-adrenergic sites. This central stimulation causes dilation of blood vessels in the periphery. Dilation of blood vessels decreases blood pressure.

Cardura and Hytrin work to block peripheral alpha-adrenergic sites which dilates blood vessels and decreases blood pressure. This action would seem to be in conflict with the way Catapres works, since Catapres stimulates alpha-adrenergic sites. The difference is that Cardura and Hytrin work on peripheral sites and Catapres works on central sites. This produces the same outcome, reduced blood pressure, but it is dependent on whether the drug works centrally or peripherally.

Common Side-Effects of these Medications

Angina (chest pain)
Hypotension
Stroke
Tachycardia (rapid heart beat)
Edema
Insomnia

Headache
Dizziness
Weakness
Fatigue
Confusion
Depression
Nervousness
Vertigo
Anxiety
Nausea
Vomiting
Diarrhea
Anorexia
Dry Mouth
Cough
Flushing
Rash
Impotence
Decreased libido
Muscle cramps
Blurred vision
Fever
Tinnitus (ringing in ears)
Arthralgia (pain in joints)
Arthritis
Flu-like symptoms

Natural Alternatives

Hawthorn – The berries of the hawthorn (*Crategus oxyacan-thoides*) have been revered since the time of the Greeks and Romans for their strengthening effects on the heart. Hawthorn lowers blood pressure by dilating blood vessels, including the cardiac arteries which feed blood to the heart muscle.

Hawthorn also produces a slowing of the heart rate which adds to the effects on blood pressure.

Coenzyme Q10 – Coenzyme Q10 (CoQ10) is essential for proper heart function and has a history of such use in Japan. As we age, or are subjected to stress, our levels of CoQ10 can diminish. This can raise our blood pressure. Supplementation with CoQ10 can decrease blood pressure by itself. Using CoQ10 should be a part of any cardiac supportive program.

Olive Leaf – The leaf of the olive (*Olea europea*) also provides a hypotensive effect. Some cultures utilized olive leaves as diuretics. Olive leaf causes increased blood flow to the heart and is also an excellent antioxidant for the cardiovascular system. The net effect of olive leaf is as a protectant (antioxidant activity) and hypotensive.

Vitamin E – Much research is being conducted at the present time on the effects of vitamin E on the heart and cardiovascular system. Vitamin E is an excellent antioxidant and seems to have particular affinity for the cardiovascular system. Like CoQ10, vitamin E should be a part of any program for cardiovascular health. Selenium, a trace element, should also be mentioned at this point. Selenium works very well with vitamin E for cardiac health.

Antioxidants – Antioxidants, such as vitamin C and the OPCs (grape seed/pine bark) should also be a part of any cardiac program. Antioxidants work on the heart and blood vessels to reduce oxidative damage. Damage to these vascular muscles can lead to hypertension. Antioxidants act as protectors of the muscle that forms the cardiovascular system.

Fish Oils, Flax Seed Oil – These oils provide omega-3 and omega-6 essential fatty acids. Essential fatty acids are required by the body to create other fatty acids. They are termed "essential" since the body cannot manufacture these fatty acids itself. Essential fatty acids have an effect on the blood, essentially in slightly thinning the blood. This provides less resistance for the heart and allows for smoother blood flow. The heart then gets blood to itself and to the other organs with more ease. Essential fatty acids would also be good at preventing blood clots from forming in the coronary arteries which leads to heart attacks.

Ginkgo – Ginkgo (*Ginkgo biloba*), like the essential fatty acids (omega-3 and 6), also acts to slightly thin the blood. This is very much like taking an aspirin per day. Many physicians suggest taking aspirin or baby aspirin each day. Aspirin also thins the blood which reduces resistance in the periphery. This lowers the load on the heart and allows blood to get to the heart muscle with more ease. Aspirin therapy is used to decrease the chance of a blood clot forming in the coronary arteries, which leads to a heart attack. Ginkgo provides the same effects on the blood.

Red Clover (*Trifolium pratense*) **and Soy –** These plants contain isoflavones which have noted but weak estrogenic activity. Estrogen has been shown to be cardioprotective. Women, once they reach menopause and decrease estrogen production, greatly increase their chance of getting heart disease. This is because of the lack of estrogen. The isoflavones are not hormones, but they do act to stimulate estrogen receptors. These compounds can provide cardioprotective effects through their actions.

B-vitamins – Supplementation with B-vitamins, particularly folic acid, B12 and B6, reduces the amount of homocysteine in the system. Homocysteine is an amino acid which has been linked to cardiovascular disease. People with genetic deficiencies in the enzymes which lower homocysteine levels die of heart attacks before age thirty. Lowering homocysteine levels is now thought to be critical. There is, unfortunately, no convenient test for homocysteine blood levels.

Coleus forskohlii – Supplementation with extracts from *Coleus forskohlii* have been shown to have hypotensive effects. Coleus works on the levels of cyclic adenosine monophosphate (cAMP) in the blood vessels, which promotes vasodilation.

L-arginine – L-arginine is an amino acid which seems to work on the nitric oxide pathway. This leads to vasodilation. L-Arginine may also inhibit platelet aggregation. This would slow the formation of a blood clot, which would decrease the risk of a heart attack, and lower blood pressure by decreasing the load on the heart muscle.

Drug/Natural Product Interactions

Care should be taken anytime one of these natural products is utilized in combination with an antihypertensive medication. Many of these natural products can have a significant impact on blood pressure which may be additive or synergistic with the medication. Lowering the blood pressure too much could lead to unwanted side effects such as dizziness. You should consult your physician and check your blood pressure often if you are adding a new supplement to your antihypertensive medication. Blood pressure cuffs for home use are recommended for those who want to keep a log of their progress and the effectiveness of their treatments.

The products which have effects on the blood, such as ginkgo and the essential fatty acids, can interact with the prescription drug Coumadin. Coumadin is a blood thinning agent which is prescribed for various reasons. You should discuss any new supplement with your physician if you are on Coumadin.

Special Considerations

Blood pressure is something that can change dramatically from minute to minute. If, overall, your blood pressure is too high, you should consider environmental factors as well as physiological factors. Lowering your salt intake often is helpful. Stress level or a simple lack of exercise can be to blame for the hypertension. Utilizing exercise and other modalities to decrease stress will also have an impact on blood pressure. This impact can be quite dramatic in many instances.

Please discuss your choice of blood pressure treatment with your physician so that he/she may monitor your progress and acquaint yourself with the acceptable levels for systolic and diastolic pressure. A diastolic value of greater than 90 mmHg is borderline as unacceptable.

Blood Pressurex
Phloestrogens

CHAPTER 13

HRT and Osteoporosis

Menopause describes a time in a woman's life when permanent cessation of the menses occurs. After menopause, a woman's hormonal balance changes. Medical science has discovered that there are many physiological events that can occur with this change in hormone balance.

One of the most important changes involves bone. Women with reduced estrogen are more prone to develop a condition called osteoporosis which is a lowering of bone mass. With reduced bone mass, the individual runs a higher risk of having broken bones, bone deformities, a stooped posture, and pain. Osteoporosis may happen to both men and women, but women are at a much greater risk since they usually have a lower bone density prior to menopause.

Another observation has been that women increase in the occurrence of heart disease after menopause. Before menopause, due to estrogen, women run a greatly reduced risk of heart disease, but after menopause they catch up to men quite quickly. This problem has also been attributed to the change in hormonal balance that occurs with menopause. Heart attacks in these women, unlike men, are often due to spasms of the coronary vessels and not coronary restrictions due to hardening of the arteries.

In an attempt to rectify this situation, the pharmaceutical

industry has developed several medications to restore the female body to premenopausal hormonal levels. The first attempt, and one still readily utilized, is to supplement with the hormone estrogen. This type of therapy, supplementing with hormones after menopause, is termed "hormone replacement therapy" or HRT.

Drugs

Premarin (conjugated estrogens)
Prempro (conjugated estrogens/medroxyprogesterone)
Estratest (estrogens/methyltestosterone)
Estraderm (estradiol transdermal)
Estrace (estradiol)
Evista (raloxifene)
Climara (estradiol transdermal)
Fosamax (alendronate)
Ogen (estropipate)
Estratab (esterified estrogens)

Fosamax and Evista, although they work in different fashions, are drugs specifically indicated for osteoporosis. Fosamax and Evista effectively stop the loss of bone. They are not considered HRT, but are included in this section due to their use in osteoporosis.

Premarin, Estraderm, Estrace, Climara, Ogen and Estratab are all various forms of estrogen. They also come in various delivery systems – most are tablets, but Climara and Estraderm are delivered as a patch that is worn on the skin. Premarin actually is derived from pregnant mare's urine (which is also where they derived the drug's name). Some of the rest of these medications are different salts of estrogen or are slightly different estrogens.

Prempro and Estratest combine both estrogens and androgens. Androgens (such as testosterone) are hormones that are usually looked at as "male" hormones. Both sexes have both androgens and estrogens. The difference is in the amounts of androgens and estrogens present – but both types of hormones are required. Progesterone is an anti-estrogenic steroid which is produced by the placenta and corpus luteum (formed at release of an egg from the ovary during ovulation). It is often referred to as the "pregnancy hormone" due to its stabilizing effect on the pregnancy. Progesterone plays an extremely important role in a woman's health, even after menopause.

It was originally assumed that simple replacement of estrogen was all that was needed by postmenopausal women. This thinking has changed in recent years. It is now understood that menopause affects not only estrogens, but also progesterone. For this reason, many physicians believe supplementing with both estrogens and progesterone is more appropriate therapy for postmenopausal women. Yet other physicians subscribe to progesterone-only therapy for postmenopausal treatment.

Common Side-Effects of These Medications

Headache
Migraine
Dizziness
Depression
Insomnia
Anxiety
Hirsutism (excess body and facial hair)
Breakthrough bleeding
Spotting
Cramps
Bloating
Nausea
Vomiting

Edema
Changes in libido
Breast pain
Breast enlargement
Hot flushes
Weight change

Natural Alternatives

Calcium and Vitamin D – It is essential to supplement with calcium to help reduce osteoporosis. Calcium is the main integral ingredient in bone. Most diets do not contain enough calcium to meet nutritional needs adequately. Calcium supplements are well tolerated and their use is highly recommended. Vitamin D, the sunshine vitamin, plays an essential role in depositing calcium and should be taken with calcium.

Dong Quai – The herb dong quai (*Angelica sinensis*) comes to us from Asia. In Asia it is considered the remedy for female complaints. Dong quai is used to relieve complaints that accompany menopause. The herb seems especially good for the treatment of hot flashes.

Black Cohosh – Black cohosh (*Cimicifuga racemosa*) has been utilized by the American Indians for centuries to relieve menstrual cramps and to alleviate the symptoms of menopause. Like dong quai, black cohosh seems particularly effective at reducing hot flashes and other conditions common to menopause.

Soy – Soy contains isoflavones which have estrogenic activity. The isoflavones of soy are not hormones, but they do stimulate estrogen receptors in the body. For this reason, a diet rich in soy products or supplements helps alleviate many of the symptoms of menopause such as osteoporosis. The estrogenic activity also is responsible for soy's reputation for cardiovascular health.

Red Clover – Like soy, red clover (*Trifolium pratense*) contains isoflavones and also has estrogenic activity. Red clover is also not a hormone, but the red clover isoflavones will stimulate estrogen receptors.

Progesterone Creams – Several companies offer creams which contain progesterone. These creams are designed to be applied to the skin, usually a sensitive area that blushes easily such as the stomach and inner thighs. The reason these areas are used is because of the abundant blood flow to those areas of skin. Once the cream is applied, some of the progesterone is absorbed into the bloodstream through the skin. Daily application of such a product creates a therapy that delivers a very low dose of progesterone to the system. This mode of therapy has proven very effective in alleviating the various complaints of menopause. Low dose topical progesterone therapy takes care of bone loss, libido, hot flashes and vaginal atrophy which can occur with menopause. Progesterone also provides protection against breast cancer and heart attacks. This is also a convenient therapy which appeals to more and more women. There have been several well-received books written on this type of therapy. If you have questions about low dose topical progesterone therapy, it is suggested that you invest in one of these books.

Care should be taken when buying a topical progesterone cream. Many companies label their products as progesterone, but in reality they only contain wild yam, soy or some other product. You should choose a reputable company that actually utilizes progesterone in their product. Try the product for a couple of months and assess the effectiveness of that product. If it is working for you then you should stick with it.

Drug/Natural Product Interactions

Any of these products has the capability of interfering with HRT. Your physician should be informed if you are utilizing one of these natural therapies.

Red clover may interfere with the prescription drug Coumadin. Coumadin is a blood-thinning agent so an interaction could be potentially serious. If you are on Coumadin, you should discuss any new therapies with your physician so that he/she may monitor your Coumadin dose.

Special Considerations

Menopause is a natural event in the life of women. Unfortunately the change in hormones can lead to several complications. Addressing these complications with a healthy diet, exercise and supplementation would seem to be a very prudent move. The natural therapies discussed here have proven quite effective for many women. You should discuss your choices with your physician.

Flash Ease

CHAPTER 14

Nausea and Vomiting

Nausea and vomiting are two very irritating conditions to those who suffer from them. Both nausea and vomiting can have several different causes. Often they are side-effects of another condition such as the flu. Other times they can be side-effects of medications being taken. Many medications can cause nausea and vomiting. Another common cause is from something we've eaten. This condition is usually referred to as food poisoning. Sometimes we can have nausea and vomiting because of anxiety about something we're about to do, such as a job interview. Morning sickness in the first trimester of pregnancy is a common occurrence. Then there is motion sickness (or vertigo) which can happen on ships, airplanes, in cars or from other causes.

Regardless of the cause, nausea and vomiting can be most unpleasant. Medically, nausea and vomiting are often treated once the underlying cause is ascertained and treated. The fact that nausea and vomiting are often signs of an underlying condition must not be overlooked. If the primary cause is being addressed, then nausea and vomiting may be treated to help alleviate that particular condition.

Nausea and vomiting have plagued man since the beginning of time. Man has, for millenia, turned to nature to help alleviate these conditions. There are several things in nature which have proven potential to help with these conditions.

Drugs

Serotonin

Kytril (granisetron)
Zofran (ondansetron)
Phenergan (promethazine)
Compazine (prochlorperazine)
Dramamine (dimenhydrinate)
Antivert (meclizine)   *other*
Scopace, Transderm-Scop (scopolamine)
Tigan (trimethobenzamide)
Marinol (dronabinol)
Reglan (metoclopramide)

Dopamine

Cause convulsions

Kytril and Zofran are from a class of drugs that affects the serotonin system. They work by being an antagonist to serotonin at a certain serotonin receptor site. These two medications are most often used in conjunction with cancer chemotherapy, which usually causes very pronounced nausea and vomiting.

Reglan, Compazine and Phenergan all work on the dopamine system in the brain. These medications seem to be particularly good at alleviating drug-induced nausea and vomiting.

Dramamine, Antivert, Scopace and Transderm-Scop are all anticholinergics. They are most effective for vertigo and motion sickness.

Marinol is actually a derivative of marijuana. This drug also works on the central nervous system but in a way different than the other drugs listed. In reality, Marinol is not utilized that much. Its use is usually restricted to chemotherapy-induced nausea and vomiting that is not responsive to other therapies.

It should also be noted that several of these medications (Dramamine, Compazine, Phenergan) are also utilized as antihistamines. They seem to be better used for nausea and vomiting because of their sedative effects. Benadryl (diphenhydramine) is another antihistamine which is sometimes employed for nausea and vomiting. The active ingredient in Benadryl is also often used in "PM" products – that is products designed to be taken at bedtime – because of its pronounced sedative effects.

Common Side-Effects of These Medications

Drowsiness
CNS depression
Rash
Restlessness
Nervousness
Insomnia
Blurred vision
Dry mouth
Dry nose
Diarrhea
Constipation
Hypotension
Confusion
Anorexia
Urinary frequency
Urinary retention
Difficult urination
Hypertension
Anxiety

Natural Alternatives

Ginger – The root of the ginger plant (*Zingiber officinale*) has been used for decades to help alleviate nausea and vomiting. Several studies have been conducted on ginger with quite favorable results.

Peppermint – Peppermint or peppermint oil is also useful for nausea and vomiting. Even chewing a piece of peppermint gum can help some individuals lessen the feelings of nausea.

Electrolytes – The term "electrolytes" refers to a group of minerals that are required for normal body function. When an individual has nausea and vomiting, the electrolytes of the body can be depleted. Many companies sell a mineral solution, or colloidal mineral solution, which can be very helpful at replenishing these lost electrolyte reserves.

Valerian – Valerian (*Valeriana officinalis*) has a slight calming effect much as the benzodiazepines (see chapter on anxiety medications). The benzodiazepines are also employed to reduce the symptoms of nausea and vomiting. Valerian can also have these types of effects.

Kava Kava – Just like valerian, the root of the kava kava (*Piper methysticum*) plant is also used as a calming sedative, much like the benzodiazepines. Kava may well provide relief of nausea and vomiting for some individuals.

Drug/Natural Product Interactions

Kava and Valerian should be used with caution if other sedative medications, such as benzodiazepines, are being used due to the possibility for over sedation. Ginger should be used with caution in individuals on Coumadin or other blood thinning therapy. Ginger has been shown to have a blood thinning effect.

Special Considerations

The underlying cause of the nausea or vomiting should not be ignored. Seek medical treatment for the cause of the nausea and vomiting and then deal with the nausea and vomiting itself.

Colloidal Minerals

CHAPTER 15

NSAIDs

Arthritis

A rthritis is a condition which afflicts millions of people. Arthritis consists of swelling and pain in a joint along with degeneration of the cartilage in the joint. The cartilage can degenerate to the point that bone ends up rubbing against bone. This type of advanced arthritis is extremely painful.

The class of pharmaceuticals created to alleviate this condition is called NSAIDs. NSAIDs stands for non-steroidal anti-inflammatory drugs. As the name implies, NSAIDs are designed to be anti-inflammatory agents. Swelling is one of the major components of arthritis, so reducing the swelling will help the pain associated with the condition. Steroids, such as prednisone, are extremely potent anti-inflammatory agents. But steroids have many unwanted side-effects. NSAIDs were developed to reduce the swelling without having the other effects that come with steroids.

One item that the NSAIDs overlooks is the degeneration of the cartilage (the cushion between bones in joints). This is a major component of the condition of arthritis. If the cartilage is nourished and given the building blocks it needs, then the joint cartilage may return back to a normal state. NSAIDs actually speed the destruction of cartilage by depriving the joint of the essential items needed to rebuild cartilage. Cartilage requires rebuilding because it is constantly being abused and damaged. This damage is normal and is normally followed by a clean-up of the damaged cartilage with rebuilding following that. If NSAIDs are introduced, this process can be cut short, resulting in ever reduced amounts of cartilage in the joint.

Drugs

n-saids

Relafen (nabumetone)
Motrin (ibuprofen)
Lodine (etodolac)
Daypro (oxaprozin)
Feldene (piroxicam)
Clinoril (sulindac)
Naprosyn (naproxen)
Voltaren (diclofenac)
Ansaid (flurbiprofen)
Nalfon (fenoprofen)
Indocin (indomethacin)
Orudis (ketoprofen)
Arthrotec (diclofenac/misoprostol)
Vioxx (rofecoxib) *cox-2 inhibitors*
Celebrex (celecoxib)

All of these drugs are considered NSAIDs: however, Vioxx and Celebrex are slightly different than the others. Both Vioxx and Celebrex are classified as COX-2 inhibitors. NSAIDs as a class work by inhibiting the synthesis of prostaglandins. Prostaglandins are important elements in several body mechanisms. One of these mechanisms is swelling and another mechanism that proves important is stomach protection. Prostaglandins help in protecting the stomach tissue from the acid produced by the stomach. This is important with NSAIDs because inhibiting prostaglandins generally will, besides reducing inflammation, also lower the stomach's ability to protect itself against the stomach acid. This leads to a very common, yet dangerous side-effect of NSAIDs – stomach ulcers.

COX-2 inhibitors were created to overcome the problem of stomach ulcers. These compounds work on a slightly different part of the prostaglandin chain. Inhibition at the COX-2 level allows for the reduction of the prostaglandins responsible for swelling while, at the same time, not affecting the prostaglandins responsible for stomach protection. In theory we then have a compound that will reduce swelling while not affecting the stomach. Unfortunately this works much better in theory than in practice. COX-2 inhibitors can also cause stomach ulcers in many cases.

Since inflammation is often a component of pain, the NSAIDs and COX-2 inhibitors are often prescribed for pain other than that caused by arthritis. These compounds are also utilized often to reduce a fever.

Common Side-Effects of these Medications

Hypertension (high blood pressure)
Blood pressure changes
Irregular heartbeat
Chest pain
Dizziness
Drowsiness
Nervousness
Fatigue
Insomnia
Tremor
Depression
Lightheadedness
Amnesia
Rash
Eczema

Menstrual disorders
Impotence
Breast pain
Heartburn
Ulcers
Indigestion
Elevated liver enzymes
Asthma
Weight increase or decrease
Leg cramps
Muscle weakness
UTI (urinary tract infections)
Difficulty breathing
Cough
Visual disturbances
Irritated eyes
Influenza-like symptoms

Natural Alternatives

Chondroitin – Chondroitin is one of the major building blocks of cartilage. Supplementation with chondroitin provides the essential components of cartilage to the joint to allow rebuilding of the cartilage.

Glucosamine – Glucosamine is also a building block of cartilage. Glucosamine is a smaller compound than chondroitin. Chondroitin is made up of glucosamine molecules. Glucosamine is one of the most effective rebuilding agents for joint cartilage.

Yucca – The yucca (*Yucca baccata*) plant has been revered for its anti-inflammatory components, believed to be the saponins.

The plant has been used by traditional herbalists to treat arthritis and other conditions of swelling.

Bromelain – This derivative from the pineapple plant also has very good anti-inflammatory properties. Bromelain may aid in reducing the swelling and pain associated with arthritis.

Morinda – The fruit of the morinda tree (*Morinda citrifolia*) is revered by the Polynesians for its ability to reduce pain and swelling. The Polynesians would utilize the ripe fruit of the morinda to treat various diseases with associated pain.

Aloe Vera – The liquid from the leaves of the aloe vera (*Aloe barbados*) has also been used to treat pain and swelling. Many people have achieved excellent pain reduction by using aloe.

Antioxidants – Supplementation with a good water-soluble antioxidant such as the OPCs (grape seed/pine bark) helps protect joint cartilage from oxidative damage which helps reduce wear. Over time, reduction of oxidative damage to cartilage can slow the degradation of the joint tissue. This would also help reduce the associated inflammation.

MSM – MSM (methylsulfonylmethane) is a substance which all humans have and require. MSM is a source of sulfur for the body. Sulfur is required in the building of cartilage. MSM has also exhibited excellent anti-inflammatory properties. Many individuals have achieved a reversal of cartilage damage by supplementation with MSM and glucosamine.

SAM-e – SAM-e (s-adenosylmethionine) is most commonly associated with the treatment of depression. SAM-e has been in use in Europe for several decades now, and it has been discovered that SAM-e plays a role in other conditions besides depression. SAM-e has been shown to help alleviate the pain associated with arthritis and aids in rebuilding the cartilage in joints. SAM-e shows great potential for application in reversing the cartilage damage associated with degenerative arthritis.

Drug/Natural Product Interactions

There are no known interactions between the NSAIDs or COX-2 inhibitors and any of the natural products listed here. It should be remembered that individuals vary and interactions are not an exact science. It could be that there are interactions that have not yet been discovered or that an individual could suffer an interaction that the general population does not have. Generally, many people have taken glucosamine, MSM and chondroitin with the NSAID or COX-2 inhibitor medications without adverse effects.

Special Considerations

It is advised that your physician be included in all components of your treatment. If you are considering using some of these natural products in conjunction with, or instead of, your prescription medication, you should advise your doctor.

Flax seed oil
omega 3

■ CHAPTER 16 ■

Pain Medications

A cute pain is a situation that all of us deal with at some time or another. The medications discussed in this chapter are all prescribed for acute pain situations. Acute pain is generally associated with some type of insult or injury to the body. Examples of acute pain for which these medications are prescribed might include surgery, injury (such as a broken bone) or migraine.

Migraine headaches are a special category of acute pain. Many individuals suffer from migraines. Migraines are extremely painful headaches that can originate from many different causes. Several medications, besides those strong medications used for acute pain, have been developed solely to deal with migraines. Some of those medications are discussed here.

Drugs

Lortab (hydrocodone/acetaminophen)
Vicodin (hydrocodone/acetaminophen)
Tylenol No. 3 (codeine/acetaminophen)
Darvocet N-100 (propoxyphene/acetaminophen)
Percocet (oxycodone/acetaminophen)
Percodan (oxycodone/aspirin)

Oxycontin (oxycodone)
Talwin (pentazocine)
Nubain (nalbuphine)
Dalgan (dezocine)
MS Contin (morphine)
Demerol (meperidine)
Dilaudid (hydromorphone)
Ultram (tramadol)
Zomig (zolmitriptan)
Maxalt (rizatriptan)
Amerge (naratriptan)
Imitrex (sumatriptan)

Narcotic analgesics

Migraine medications

Zomig, Maxalt, Amerge and Imitrex are all part of a new class of medication known as serotonin receptor agonists. These compounds are specific for a very certain type of serotonin receptor. Their function is to stimulate this special serotonin receptor. They are prescribed for migraine headaches. It has been discovered that these special serotonin receptors play a part in some people's migraine headaches. For those individuals, these drugs have proven very effective.

Ultram is a relatively new medication whose mechanism of action is not completely understood. It is known that Ultram works within the central nervous system and has some pain relieving effects like narcotics (see below) but without many of the other effects. Ultram is usually prescribed for people with chronic (long-term) pain. This would be beneficial for those suffering from arthritis or other pain of a chronic nature.

The rest of the medications listed above are considered narcotic analgesics. The narcotics work directly on the central nervous system to decrease pain impulses going to the brain. These compounds are extremely potent and can cause addiction and impairment of cognitive functions. Some of these medications are narcotic analgesics mixed with another medication such as aspirin or acetaminophen. In these medications the patient achieves central pain relief from the narcotic and peripheral pain relief through the prostaglandin system from the aspirin or acetaminophen.

Common Side-Effects of these Medications

Respiratory depression
Bradycardia (slow heart rate)
Lightheadedness
Dizziness
Sedation
Nausea
Vomiting
Sweating
Flushing
Faintness
Tachycardia (rapid heart rate)
Euphoria
Delirium
Insomnia
Headache
Agitation
Anxiety
Hallucinations
Drowsiness
Disorientation
Blurred vision
Amnesia
Lethargy
Diarrhea
Cramps
Abdominal pain
Dry mouth

Hives
Rash
Dependency

Natural Alternatives

DL-Phenylalanine – The amino acid phenylalanine can help alleviate significant pain. L-phenylalanine, which is the amino acid normally utilized by the body, is the beginning point for several neurotransmitters such as epinephrine and norepinephrine. These neurotransmitters play an important role in reducing the perception of pain.

D-phenylalanine, which is produced along with L-phenylalanine, is also useful for pain. D-phenylalanine has been shown to have direct effect on the central nervous system to reduce pain perception. This is much the same as the narcotic analgesics. D-phenylalanine, however, does not manifest the complex of adverse effects that the narcotic analgesics do.

Morinda – The morinda tree fruit (*Morinda citrifolia*) is revered by the Polynesian people for its ability to relieve pain. The ripened fruit is often applied directly to a wound or sore area to relieve the pain. Morinda may also be taken internally for the same purpose.

Willow – The bark from willow trees (*Salix spp.*) such as white willow, purple willow and black willow, contain glycosides of salicyl alcohol and salicylates. Salicylates have activity much like aspirin which is a salicylate derivative. Salicylates aid in reducing fever, inflammation and pain.

SAM-e – SAM-e (s-adenosylmethionine) is a substance present in all human beings. SAM-e as a supplement has only recently come to press. The compound has been used in

Europe since the 1960s. SAM-e is usually associated with the relief of depression. SAM-e works very well for depression, but it also works in other areas. Since SAM-e may have an effect on the central nervous system neurotransmitter serotonin, it could be of benefit to individuals who suffer from serotonin sensitive migraines. SAM-e would be taken on a daily basis to prevent the onset of migraines.

St. John's Wort – St. John's Wort (*Hypericum perforatum*), like SAM-e, may help individuals who suffer from migraine. St. John's Wort may help establish consistent brain levels of some neurotransmitters which could prevent the onset of migraines.

Feverfew – Feverfew (*Chrysanthemum parthenium*) has been utilized by herbalists for centuries to treat individuals suffering from migraines. One active ingredient in feverfew, parthenolide, seems also to have an effect on brain levels of serotonin. This is reported to be the mechanism of action in utilizing feverfew to prevent migraines. Feverfew should be taken on a daily basis by those who suffer from migraines to prevent the onset of a migraine.

Drug/Natural Product Interactions

There are no known interactions with these natural products and any of the prescription medications listed. Care should be used, however, when using one of the migraine medications that are serotonin agonists along with a natural product (SAM-e, St. John's Wort and feverfew) which also affect serotonin levels in the brain.

Natural products which cause drowsiness, such as kava kava and valerian, may increase the drowsiness of the narcotic analgesics. Care should be taken when combining these therapies.

Special Considerations

Pain is generally an indicator of a larger problem. Please consult your physician if you have acute pain or suffer from frequent migraines to determine if there is a more extensive problem.

Nature's Phenyltol

Migraine
use Gastro Health

CHAPTER 17

Prostate

The prostate is a doughnut shaped gland found at the base of the bladder in males. The urethra (the tube that leads from the bladder and discharges urine to the outside) goes through the "doughnut hole" of the prostate. The prostate is important in male sexual function, providing part of the seminal fluid required for reproduction.

With advancing age in men, the prostate often becomes inflamed and swollen. Sometimes this swelling can be due to prostate cancer. If this is the case, the prostate is usually surgically removed, although there are new methods being developed for removing the prostate without surgery. Prostate cancer can usually be detected by a blood test for elevated levels of prostate specific antigen (PSA).

If the prostate is not cancerous, yet there is swelling, the condition is known as BPH (benign prostatic hypertrophy). BPH causes urinary frequency and difficult urination. Often a man will need to urinate, but will be unable to due to the swelling of the prostate around the urethra.

There are several medications which have been developed to aid men with BPH.

Drugs

Flomax (tamsulosin)
Hytrin (terazosin)
Cardura (doxazosin)
Proscar (finasteride)

Flomax, Hytrin and Cardura all belong to a class of drugs known as antiadrenergic agents. These drugs block the alpha-1 adrenergic receptors. This causes two things which are of clinical importance. First, there is a dramatic lowering of blood pressure. Many may recognize one of these medications as their blood pressure medication. Lowering blood pressure is the most recognized effect of most of these medications. The second effect of clinical significance, however, is reduction of BPH symptoms. This is achieved by blocking the same receptors as those affecting blood pressure.

Proscar is a different class of medication. This drug works by affecting the conversion of testosterone to dihydrotestosterone (DHT) and on receptors on the prostate that are sensitive to testosterone and DHT. This mechanism of action also alleviates the symptoms of BPH. It is of interest to note that the active ingredient of Proscar, finasteride, is also marketed as a hair growth drug under the name Propecia. Only the strength of the tablet has been changed.

Common Side-Effects of these Medications

Tachycardia (rapid heart rate)
Hypotension
Diarrhea
Nausea
Vomiting
Dry mouth
Flu-like symptoms

Joint pain
Dizziness
Depression
Drowsiness
Nervousness
Impotence
Urinary frequency
Headache
Edema
Weight gain
Tinnitus (ringing in ears)
Blurred vision
Nasal congestion
Constipation
Erectile dysfunction
Decreased libido

Natural Alternatives

Saw Palmetto – The berry of the saw palmetto (*Serenoa repens*) has been utilized for the condition of BPH for generations. Recent scientific study of the berry and its active ingredients has shown a pharmacology similar to that of Proscar (which, by the way, is the best tolerated of the above medications for BPH). Saw palmetto also seems to work on the conversion of testosterone to DHT and on receptors in the prostate. Several head-to-head studies with Proscar have shown equal effects on the symptoms of BPH, but the saw palmetto group usually achieves the end results sooner than the drug group. The saw palmetto group also experiences fewer side-effects than the drug group.

Stinging Nettle – The leaves of the stinging nettle (*Urtica dioica*) have traditionally also been used to treat symptoms associated with BPH. More modern research has suggested that this benefit may be due to the activities of stinging nettle active ingredients on certain enzyme functions of the prostate. The herb has shown benefit in treating BPH.

Zinc – The element zinc is vitally important to the prostate. Zinc supplementation should be included in any program designed for prostate health.

Soy and Red Clover – Both soy and red clover (*Trifolium pratense*) have estrogenic effects. Estrogen is the hormone that counteracts testosterone. Incorporating a diet that is rich in soy-based foods could help alleviate the symptoms of BHP.

Pygeum – The bark of the pygeum (*Prunus africana*) has been utilized for BPH. European studies have shown great promise for this natural product in the treatment of BPH. The mechanism of action probably involves some of pygeum's active ingredients – the phytosterols.

Drug/Natural Product Interactions

Care should be taken when combining therapies that have similar mechanisms of action, such as Proscar with saw palmetto. Although there is no known direct interaction between the two, there is more of a chance of this happening since both compounds are working on the same sites.

If you are on Flomax, Hytrin or Cardura, you should be careful when using natural products that reduce blood pressure (see chapter on high blood pressure medications). Flomax, Hytrin and Cardura can all have a significant impact on lowering blood pressure, so adding a natural product that reduces blood pressure may cause too much of a reduction in pressure.

Special Considerations

Saw palmetto, Pygeum and Stinging Nettle may all interfere with the standard PSA test given to determine prostate function. If you are using one of these natural products and your doctor suggests a PSA test, you should tell him/her about the natural product. The test may still be performed, but you will need to go for a time without taking the supplement before having the PSA administered.

Men's Formula
Pygeum
Phytoestrogens

CHAPTER 18

Sleep Medications

Sleep is something that sometimes eludes us. Often we find ourselves thinking about the day's activities or some problem in our lives, and we just can't get to sleep. If we go without sleep for too long, then that begins to wear on us. Sleep deprivation can adversely affect our lives by interfering with our jobs, school, home, etc., and taken to extreme it results in depressive neurosis.

As with other conditions, sleeplessness is often a sign of something else that is occurring. Sleeplessness can be treated, but the underlying cause of the sleeplessness should be determined and dealt with. If an individual is under too much stress, then something should be done about that. Likewise, if a person is not getting sleep because of depression, then the depression should be addressed. If you suffer from chronic sleeplessness, it is advised that you contact a physician that deals with sleep disorders to help ascertain the exact reason for the sleeplessness.

The pharmaceutical industry has many medications in its arsenal to alleviate sleeplessness. All work on the central nervous system in one way or another. Possibly the most common sleep medications are the shorter acting benzodiazepines. Also utilized often for sleeplessness are the barbiturates, which are an older class of medication that are very successful but habit-forming.

Drugs

Prosom (estazolam)
Restoril (temazepam)
Ambien (zolpidem)
Dalmane (flurazepam)
Doral (quazepam)
Placidyl (ethchlorvynol)
Sonata (zaleplon)
Halcion (triazolam)
Unisom (doxylamine)
Nytol (diphenhydramine)
Mebaral (mephobarbital)
Seconal (secobarbital)
Nembutal (pentobarbital)

Nembutal, Seconal and Mebaral are all of the barbiturate class. The barbiturates are very sedating and are often used in conjunction with anesthesia and surgery.

Prosom, Restoril, Dalmane, Doral and Halcion are all considered benzodiazepines. They all are short acting, so their intent is to cause pronounced drowsiness and then wear off before morning.

Ambien, Placidyl and Sonata are all considered nonbarbiturate sedative/hypnotics. They are not related to either the benzodiazepines or the barbiturates. They usually work on the gamma aminobutyric acid (GABA) system in the brain, much like the benzodiazepines. The GABA system is an inhibitor of the nervous system. GABA calms down the nervous system and causes relaxation.

Unisom and Nytol (along with many other diphenhydramine compounds) are over the counter medications which are designed to help with short term sleeplessness. They are classified as antihistamines, but they have a great deal of drowsiness associated with their use. It is the drowsiness that is marketed as an over the counter sleep aid.

Common Side-Effects of these Medications

Bradycardia (slow heart rate)
Tachycardia (rapid heart rate)
Hypertension
Hypotension
Edema
Sedation
Depression
Lethargy
Fatigue
Lightheadedness
Memory impairment
Confusion
Amnesia
Stupor
Slurred speech
Euphoria
Irritability
Skin rash
Diarrhea
Constipation
Dry mouth
Change in libido
Change in appetite
Visual disturbances
Dependency

Natural Alternatives

B-vitamins – The B-vitamins are essential for proper nervous system function. An individual under stress requires more B-vitamins than usual due to the extra need by the CNS. Having the proper amount of B-vitamins in the system may help reduce stress and allow sufficient relaxation to induce sleep.

Kava Kava – Kava Kava (*Piper methysticum*) has active ingredients that work much the same as the benzodiazepines. Kava works on the GABA system of the brain to create relaxation and causes drowsiness. Kava, taken at bedtime, works quite well to help with periods of sleeplessness.

Valerian – Like kava, Valerian (*Valeriana officinalis*) also seems to have its effects on the GABA system in the brain. Valerian helps the nervous system calm down and allows sleep to come more easily

Co Enzyme Q10 (CoQ10) – Like the B-vitamins, CoQ10 is also required by the brain and central nervous system. Deficiencies of CoQ10 can manifest themselves in different ways, sleeplessness being one possible way.

Melatonin – Melatonin is a natural compound produced by the pineal gland in the brain. Melatonin seems to be responsible for our sleep/wake pattern. Supplementation with melatonin tells the brain that it is time to sleep. This natural product is very effective in inducing sleep. Many people praise melatonin for aiding in reducing jet lag.

Drug/Natural Product Interactions

Care should be used when mixing together any sleep agents—whether or not they are natural or prescription. Mixing sleep agents can lead to over sedation or coma. If you are on a prescription sleep aid and wish to try a natural alternative, you should contact your physician for the proper way to discontinue the prescription sleep aid.

Special Considerations

Many of the prescription sleep aids, especially some of the benzodiazepines and the barbiturates, can be seriously habit-forming. For this reason, it is not advisable to discontinue suddenly the use of a prescription sleep aid that has been used for some time. Your physician can help instruct you in the best way to taper off of your prescription medication.

Snor-Ease

(3) drops of Lavender in bath water

CHAPTER 19

Thyroid

One of the most commonly treated conditions involving pharmaceuticals is hypothyroidism (low thyroid function). Some people may suffer from hyperthyroidism (high thyroid function), but this condition is usually treated by surgery, radiation, or chemical removal of the thyroid. The patient is then in a hypothyroid situation, which has to be treated pharmaceutically.

The thyroid secretes a hormone, called T4, which is then converted into T3. T3 is largely responsible for our basal metabolic rate. The body utilizes T3 to keep the fires of metabolism burning. If a person is hypothyroid, they are usually heavy (due to low use of calories) and have a lack of energy. Thyroid replacement therapy counteracts this by supplying the body with the T3 hormone or a mixture of T3 and T4 hormone.

Drugs

Armour Thyroid (thyroid desiccated)
Synthroid (levothyroxine)
Levoxyl (levothyroxine)
Thyrolar (liotrix)

Armour Thyroid is composed of desiccated animal thyroid glands. This provides both T4 and T3 to the body.

Thyrolar is a synthetic mixture of T4 and T3 which supplements the body according to the natural mixture of T4 to T3.

Synthroid and Levoxyl directly supplement synthetic T4.

Common Side-Effects of these Medications

Palpitations (irregular pulse of the heart)
Tachycardia (rapid heart beats)
Arrhythmias (irregular heart beat)
Angina (chest pain)
Allergic reaction
Tremors
Headache
Nervousness
Insomnia
Diarrhea
Vomiting
Weight loss
Menstrual irregularities
Sweating
Heat intolerance
Fever

Natural Alternatives

Kelp – Kelp, which is a giant seaweed, is utilized in cases of thyroid insufficiency (hypothyroidism) because of its high iodine content. The thyroid requires iodine to make T4 hormone. Iodine is an integral component in both T3 and T4. Supplementation with this iodine helps support the thyroid as it produces T4.

Capsicum – Capsicum (*Capsicum annuum*) has been utilized by herbalists for centuries to nourish and support the thyroid function.

Irish Moss – Like kelp, Irish moss (*Chondrus crispus*) contains a high percentage of iodine. Iodine is essential to thyroid function.

7-Keto DHEA – There is a patented product, utilized for weight loss, which is called 7-keto DHEA. DHEA (dehydroepiandrosterone) is a hormone precursor produced by the adrenal glands. 7-keto DHEA is a common metabolite of DHEA. The 7-keto metabolite seems to be responsible for increasing the amount of free T3 in the system. The patented product is usually sold as a weight loss aid, since 7-keto DHEA increases T3. Increased levels of T3 would raise basal metabolic rate, which would cause a weight loss. 7-keto DHEA may be of benefit to those with hypothyroidism since it raises levels of T3. Some thyroid function would be required in order for 7-keto DHEA to work.

Drug/Natural Product Interactions

Stimulant products, such as synephrine and ephedrine, may cause too much stimulation for an individual taking thyroid replacement hormones. You should consult your physician if you are on one of these medications and wish to use synephrine or ephedrine.

Special Considerations

If you are taking any product to supplement your thyroid function, you should consult your physician to have your thyroid function evaluated periodically. This would include drugs for thyroid or natural products for thyroid function.

Thyroid Activator
Master Gland

■ CHAPTER 20 ■

Ulcers and Hyperacidity

Ulcers, hyperacidity (excess acid production in the stomach) and GERD (gastroesophageal reflux disease – commonly referred to as "heart burn") are common problems that plague our modern society. It seems that, for most of us, our comfortable lifestyle is chewing up our stomachs.

Hyperacidity and GERD both have the majority of their roots in our lifestyles. Consuming too much food, being overweight, lack of exercise, caffeine consumption and high fat foods are contributing factors. Add to these the stresses of work and a too busy personal life and you have the makings for heartburn and hyperacidity.

Ulcers can be caused by drugs (see particularly the chapter on NSAIDs) or by too much acid finally getting to the lining of the stomach. In addition, it has recently been discovered that a certain bacterium, Helicobacter pylori (or H. pylori for short), seems to be at least partially responsible for many ulcers. For this reason many physicians will treat an ulcer with a course of antibiotics (see the chapter on antibiotics). This type of therapy has proven effective for *H. pylori* ulcers.

Drugs

H2 antagonists

Zantac (ranitidine)
Pepcid (famotidine)
Axid (nizatidine)
Tagamet (cimetidine)
Prilosec (omeprazole)   *Proton pump inhibitors*
Prevacid (lansoprazole)
Aciphex (rabeprazole)
Protonix (pantoprazole)

Zantac, Pepcid, Axid and Tagamet are all of a class of drugs called H2 antagonists. They block a certain histamine receptor which is present on the gastric parietal cells. This blockage reduces gastric acid secretions.

Prilosec, Prevacid, Aciphex and Protonix are the new generation of stomach medicines. They are from a class of drugs termed proton pump inhibitors (or PPIs). PPIs completely block the enzyme system which secretes acid into the stomach. This means that all acid production in the stomach is curtailed.

Common Side-Effects of these Medications

Headache
Fatigue
Dizziness
Confusion
Agitation
Anxiety
Depression
Insomnia
Rash
Nausea

Vomiting
Diarrhea
Constipation
Abdominal discomfort
Loss of libido
Impotence
Allergic reaction
Angina (chest pain)
Bradycardia (slow heart beat)
Vertigo
Tremors
Amnesia
Acne

Natural Alternatives

Calcium antacids – Several companies make an antacid from natural calcium sources. The calcium salt neutralizes the acid in the stomach. This takes the stomach from a hyperacid state to a more normal acid state.

Ginger – Ginger (*Zingiber officinale*) has often been used to alleviate stomach discomforts. Ginger stimulates the stomach to empty its contents into the small intestines sooner. This moves the food down the digestive tract and out of the stomach. As this food moves out of the stomach, the acid will be reduced and the likelihood of acid backing up into the esophagus (which is more likely with food present in the stomach) to cause GERD is greatly reduced.

Capsicum – Capsicum (*Capsicum annuum*) is a traditional folk cure for ulcers. Herbalists have utilized this compound for years to treat ulcers and stomach discomforts.

Pau d'Arco and Clove – Both Pau d'Arco (*Tabebuia heptaphylla*) and clove (*Eugenia aromatica*) have active compounds that have shown specific activity against H. *pylori*. These products may be effective against ulcers which have the H. pylori component.

B-Vitamins – B-vitamins help reduce some of the effects of stress by feeding the nervous system. Since stomach problems such as ulcers and hyperacidity can be caused by too much stress, B-vitamins may be of benefit in reducing that stress.

Antioxidants – Antioxidants, such as OPCs (grape seed/pine bark) can be utilized to reduce wear on the stomach and to protect the nervous system from stress damage.

Drug/Natural Product Interactions

Ginger may interact with the anticoagulant drug Coumadin. Care should be taken in using ginger if Coumadin is prescribed.

Special Considerations

Ulcers and hyperacidity, like many other conditions, are usually the results of some other factors. Lifestyle, stress levels and underlying diseases should be assessed. Often times these problems with the stomach may be alleviated by addressing our stress level or some other problem.

Gastro Health
stomach comfort

CHAPTER 21

Other Medications

There are many other prescription medications available. The scope of this book has not been to list every prescription medication – only some of those most commonly prescribed. The medications listed in this chapter are also commonly prescribed. They did not, however, neatly fit in any of the other chapters. In an attempt to be more complete, a discussion of some of these medications is included in this chapter.

K-Dur, Klor-Con (Potassium)

These medications are potassium supplements. They simply restore potassium levels to the body. Some of the medications we've discussed such as Lasix (see chapter on diuretics) can significantly decrease levels of potassium in the system. A prescription drug such as K-Dur is often prescribed along with Lasix to resupply the body's potassium levels.

Natural Alternatives

Potassium levels can often be controlled with diet. Many foods, such as bananas, are high in potassium. Often this is all that is needed to re-establish potassium levels. Alternatively,

Juniper berries, uva ursi and dandelion are all excellent sources of potassium. Work with your physician to check your potassium levels and therapy choice.

Soma (carisoprodol), Lioresal (baclofen) and Flexeril (cyclobenzaprine)

These compounds are all skeletal muscle relaxants. Many people suffer from muscle spasms due to an injury or some other cause. These medications relax the skeletal muscle to stop the spasms.

Natural Alternatives

Possibly the best natural muscle relaxant is kava kava. Kava kava causes a general relaxation which includes relaxing skeletal smooth muscle. Kava can cause drowsiness, so care should be taken with its use.

Viagra (sildenafil)

This drug has become a blockbuster. Viagra is prescribed for erectile dysfunction in men. It works on the nitric oxide system to dilate blood vessels in the penis.

Natural Alternatives

Ginkgo – *Ginkgo biloba* has a slight thinning effect on the blood. This allows more blood flow to the male genitalia which may help with erectile dysfunction.

Yohimbe – The yohimbe (*Pausinystalia yohimbe*) has been utilized for centuries to treat erectile dysfunction. Yohimbe works to dilate blood vessels and increase blood flow to the genitalia.

L-Arginine – This amino acid also works on the nitric oxide pathway and has the effect to relax blood vessels and increase blood flow.

Dilantin (phenytoin), Depakote (valproic acid), Depakene (valproic acid), Tegretol (carbamazepine), Neurontin (gabapentin)

These medications are classified as anticonvulsants. They are usually prescribed for seizure disorders such as epilepsy. They usually work in some way to raise the level of stimulus required to cause a seizure. This action is termed "raising the seizure threshold."

Natural Alternatives

It should be remembered that seizure disorders can be very serious. Your physician should be included in any therapy choices you make so that he/she may monitor your progress.

Kava Kava – Kava kava (*Piper methysticum*) works on the GABA system to cause relaxation. The mechanism of action of the kavalactones (the active ingredients in kava) is very similar to those of the benzodiazepines. The benzodiazepines are also used as anticonvulsants.

Valerian – Valerian (*Valeriana officinalis*) is also used for its relaxing qualities. Valerian may prove of benefit to some suffering from seizure disorders.

GABA – Several companies offer gamma aminobutyric acid (GABA). GABA is the neurotransmitter that works on the inhibitory nervous system. This is the system that the benzodiazepines work on to cause relaxation. Supplementation with GABA would also produce this effect.

Antioxidants – Antioxidants should be used to protect the central nervous system from oxidative damage.

Coenzyme Q10 – CoQ10 is vitally important for proper CNS function. CoQ10 supplementation with a seizure disorder is highly recommended.

Coumadin (Warfarin)

Coumadin is a blood-thinning agent. It is prescribed for many different reasons. Generally it is prescribed to prevent growth of a blood clot formed in a vein, such as in the leg. These clots, often called DVTs (deep vein thrombosis) are relatively common and are usually treated with Coumadin. Coumadin may then be prescribed to prevent future DVTs.

Natural Alternatives

Fish Oil, Flax Seed Oil – These oils have a thinning effect on the blood. This effect may be enough to prevent DVTs.

Ginkgo – Ginkgo (*Ginkgo biloba*) is an excellent blood-thinning agent. Ginkgo supplementation may also be enough to prevent DVTs.

NOTE: Coumadin therapy should not be taken lightly. Do not discontinue Coumadin without consulting your physician. You should also consult your physician if you are on Coumadin and considering taking any new supplements. Anything upsetting the normal absorption of vitamin K (the coagulation vitamin) or its function in the production of blood clotting factors in the liver must be avoided. Mineral oil laxatives, antibiotics, and vitamin K as a supplement are all examples. Your doctor will want to run tests when you start a new supplement to make sure there is not an interaction with the Coumadin and, if there is, to adjust the Coumadin dosage.

Many different things interact with Coumadin. Obviously the alternative products listed above may cause too much blood thinning if combined with Coumadin. In addition, some natural products that are known to have interactions with Coumadin include: ginger, garlic, ginseng, ginkgo, flax seed oil and fish oil. There are many other natural products that are suspected. You should consult your physician or pharmacist whenever you are considering taking a new supplement to check for known interactions. You should consult your physician whenever you begin a new supplement so that testing may be done to make sure there is no interaction with the Coumadin and, if there is an interaction, that the Coumadin dose be properly adjusted.

Deltasone (prednisone), Celestone (betamethasone), Decadron (dexamethasone), Cortef (hydrocortisone), Medrol (methylprednisolone)

These agents are classified as glucocorticoids. They work on the adrenocorticoid system. Naturally occurring adrenocorticoid steroids have anti-inflammatory and salt-retaining properties. The steroids that have anti-inflammatory properties are the glucocorticoids. These glucocorticoids are extremely potent anti-inflammatories. They are usually prescribed for conditions that include swelling such as severe arthritis.

Natural Alternatives

Methylsulfonylmethane – Methylsulfonylmethane (MSM) is a naturally occurring compound that contains sulfur. Sulfur is essential in many body functions and structures. MSM has been shown effective against arthritis because of its anti-inflammatory properties.

*See also the chapter on NSAIDs.

NOTE: There is no natural product that does exactly what prednisone will do. It should be ascertained what the prednisone is being used for and then tailor therapy to achieve that outcome. People on prednisone should supplement with a B-vitamin complex, vitamin C, zinc and magnesium to offset the effect prednisone is having on the adrenal glands.

References

The bulk of this book is written from the author's own personal experience. There are, however, several references that the author utilizes consistently. These references have been invaluable in the preparation of this book.

Fetrow, C.W.; Avila, J.R. Professional's Handbook of Complimentary and Alternative Medicines. Springhouse, PA: Springhouse Corporation. 1999.

Brinker, F. Herb Contraindications and Drug Interactions. Second Ed. Sandy, OR: Eclectic Medical Publications. 1998.

The Lawrence Review of Natural Products. St. Louis, MO: Facts and Comparisons. 2001.

Duke, J.A. CRC Handbook of Medicinal Herbs. Boca Raton, FL: CRC Press, Inc. 1985.

Murray, M.; Pizzorno, J. Encyclopedia of Natural Medicine. Second Ed. Rocklin, CA: Prima Publishing. 1998.

Tyler, V.E. Herbs of Choice. New York, NY: Pharmaceutical Products Press. 1994.

Tyler, V.E. The Honest Herbal. New York, NY: Pharmaceutical Products Press. 1993.

Drug Facts and Comparisons. St. Louis, MO: Facts and Comparisons. 2000.

The Green Book. Pleasant Grove, UT: Woodland Publishing. 1997.

Newall, C.A.; Anderson, L.A.; Phillipson, J.D. Herbal Medicines: A Guide for Health-Care Professionals. London, England: The Pharmaceutical Press. 1996.

Robbers, J.E.; Speedie, M.K.; Tyler, V.E. Pharmacognosy and Pharmacobiotechnology. Baltimore, MD: Williams and Wilkins. 1996.

Steadman's Medical Dictionary. 26th Ed. Baltimore, MD: Williams and Wilkins. 1995.

The Merck Index. Twelfth Ed. Whitehouse Station, NJ: Merck and Company. 1996.

Miller, L.G.; Murray, W.J. [Eds.] Herbal Medicinals: A Clinician's Guide. Binghamton, NY: Pharmaceutical Products Press. 1998.

Index

About The Author

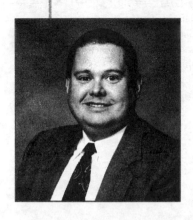

Clell M. Fowles is a 1990 graduate of the University of Utah College of Pharmacy in Salt Lake City, Utah. He earned a Bachelor of Science degree in Pharmacy and Medicinal Chemistry. He has been involved in pharmacy for over 15 year and has experience in hospital, home health, nuclear, and retail pharmacy.

Mr. Fowles also has a Bachelor of Arts degree from Utah State University in Logan, Utah. His degree from Utah State is in History with a minor in Sociology.

He is currently Manager of Health Sciences with a leading natural product company based in Provo, Utah. His work revolves around educating people about prescription medications and the role of natural products in people's health. He is a strong advocate of natural healing.

In addition to this book, Mr. Fowles has also lectured and spoken across the country on various health topics. He is recognized as an expert in prescription medications and natural remedies and is a much sought after speaker.

Order Form

To order more copies of *Drugs and Natural Alternatives*, please fill out this form and mail it to:

DAC Health
138 East 12300 South Ste C. #183
Draper, Utah 84020-7965

Please make check payable to: DAC Health

Quantity: _____
Price Each (See Price List): _____
Subtotal: _____
Utah Residents add 6.6% Sales Tax: _____
Shipping and Handling (See Table): _____
Total Enclosed
(U.S. funds. Check, Cash or Money Order): $ _____

Pricing:
1-3 Copies: $15.95 Each
4-10 Copies: $14.25 Each
11+ Copies: $13.00 Each

Shipping & Handling:
1-3 Copies: $2.50
4-10 Copies: $4.50
11+ Copies: $5.50

Name _____

Mailing/Shipping Address _____

_____

_____

Phone _____

email _____

Please allow 4-8 weeks for delivery.